Other Books By The Auth

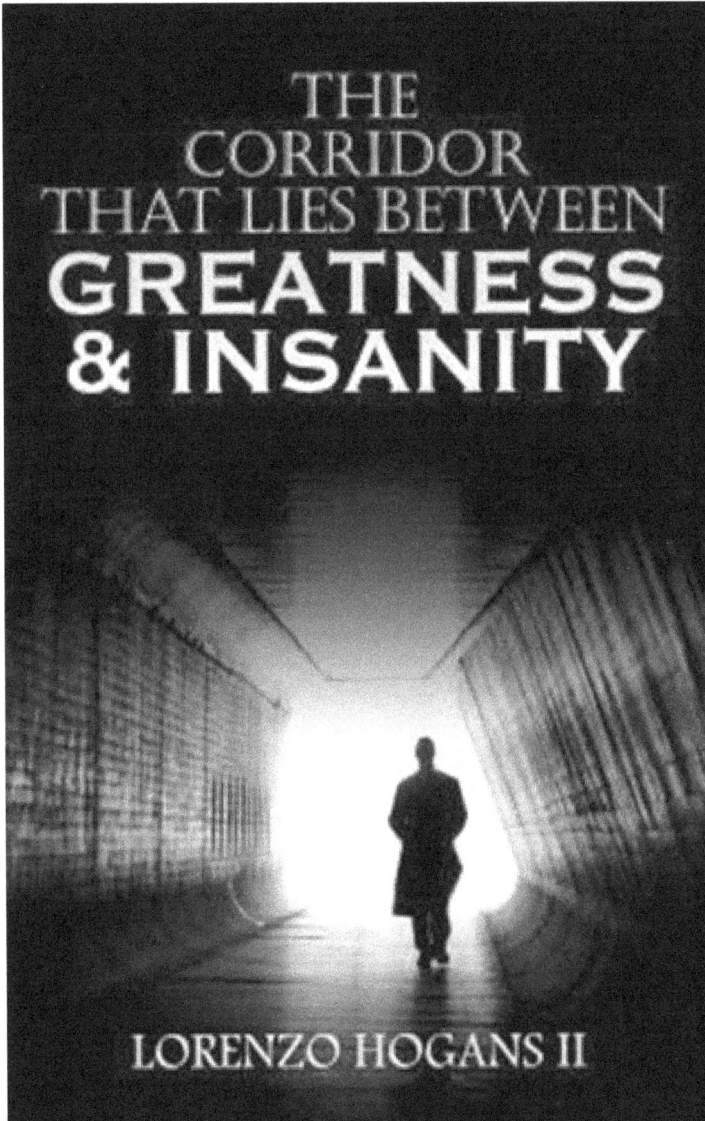

THE CORRIDOR THAT LIES BETWEEN GREATNESS & INSANITY

LORENZO HOGANS II

-A spiritual memoir on how to deal with struggle God's way and bounce back from destruction

Available on Amazon.com

PARAMEDIC

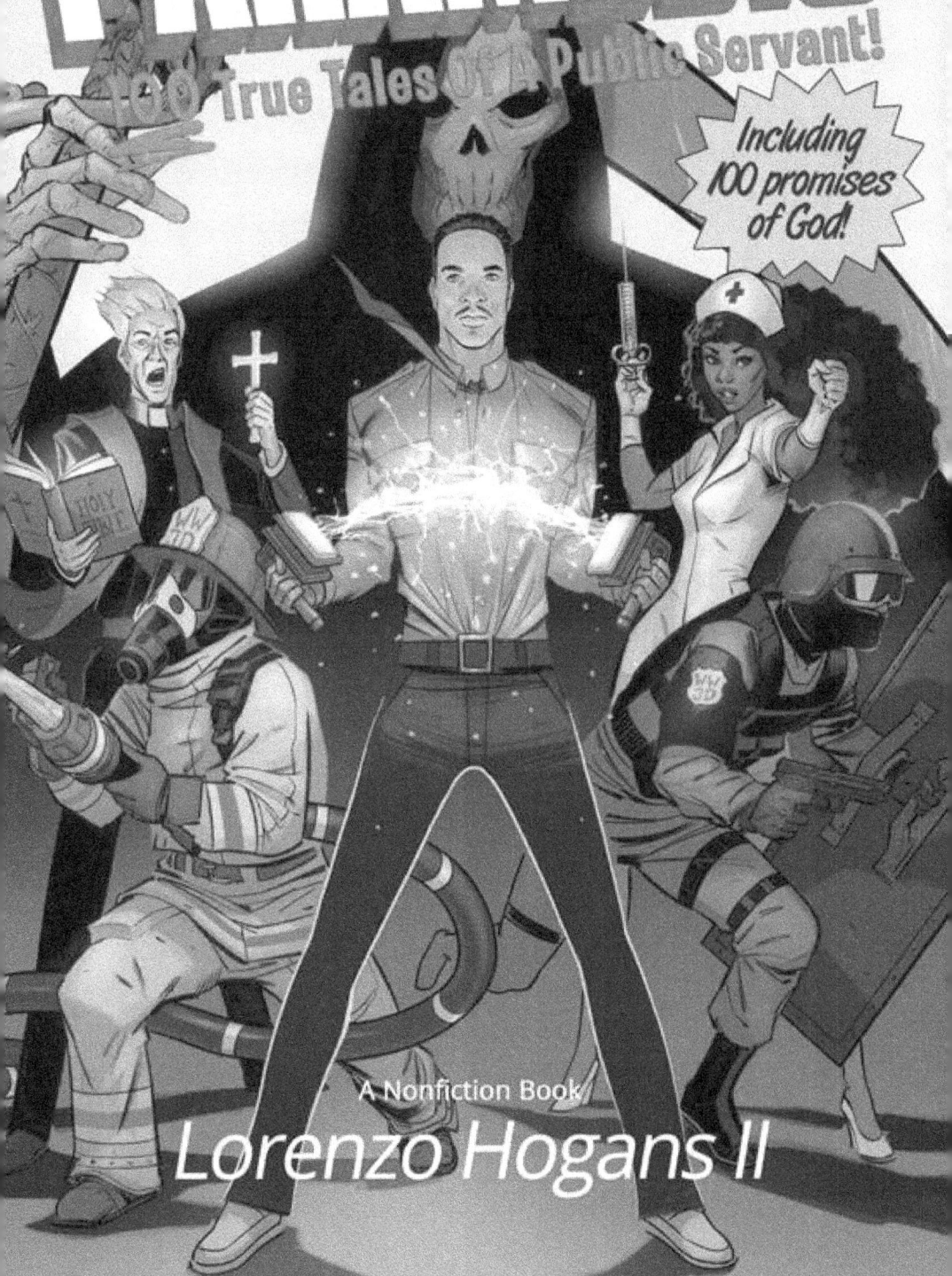

ISBN-13: 9780996397513
ISBN-10: 0996397515

This book is dedicated to everyone, no exclusions necessary.

Life and the gospel are comparable to a scary movie. When you watch a scary movie, there always seems to be that character trying to tell the other characters of a truth that seems too farfetched to believe and so it is swept under the rug. Life is a scary movie itself; it can be a real terror. The gospel is that forewarning of truth that may be a stretch to believe and I am but a character in the real world urging you to believe in God's promises... — and you must— before it's too late... because when your destiny is sealed, it is for all eternity.

Table of Contents

Acknowledgments

Don't be fooled by what you've been conditioned to identify as a hero on television or comic books. Real-life heroes don't wear capes or have super-powers. No, the real heroes are the men and women who get out there every day, work hard and strive to take care of their families. In light of this truth, the cover art of this book is a tribute to those everyday heroes. I apologize in advance for not being able to depict every kind of everyday hero, but don't think you have been forgotten. To the single-parent persevering to make ends meet: you are a true hero. To the bus driver safely ensuring that that group of kids gets to school safely: you are a hero. To the person who never gets acknowledged for the job they do, even though it irrefutably benefits others: you too are a true hero.

We all are, or at least have been given the potential to become one by contributing our God-given talents to society. Thank you to everyone who doesn't hold their contributions back, whether large or small. I believe the world is much more harmonious when we all participate in love. It's like a great orchestra. God is the master of ceremonies waving his wand up at the front of the stage and we, the musicians, can choose to play our instruments (gifts) in or out of sync. An individual who deserves an exceptional applaud is German Garcia, my cover artist, who did such a breathtaking job on the cover art. German illustrated many comic books for *Marvel Comics* and I consider it a blessing from God to have been able to collaborate with such a powerhouse artist. Finally, I'd like to acknowledge my Lord and Savior. You are the tenacity within my bones, the love within my heart and the reason for my existence. Let all things I do be for your glory.

Prologue

So you're sitting in your car, cruising down the street, when out of nowhere a giant cube on wheels bombards your personal space with an offensively loud air horn, flickering red lights and screaming sirens. It's time to get out of the way; you either freeze up and stay where you are, or you make haste to swerve to the left or to the right. This big box on wheels has just invaded your path of travel and now that it has passed you by, you check your mirrors in each location of your vehicle and proceed to ease back into the normal flow of traffic. Off into the distance the ambulance goes, speeding down the street to its destination. It is evident that an emergency has arisen – someone needs help. But have you ever thought of just where on earth that ambulance ends up? What kind of emergency is taking place? Whether or not that person will be okay? Or how about the God-awful thought that a family member or loved one is involved?

I'm Lorenzo, one of the paramedics that zoom by in an emergency and I'm here to share with you what happens after the loud ambulance passes you. Maybe later things will be different, but today I carry a *thorn* in my side, metaphorically speaking. The thought of it burdens me slightly on each call, but I manage it well thanks to the Lord. My would-be wife decided to become a pole dancer (stripper) and unfortunately that's a form of work I couldn't stand for. I wrote about that painful ordeal in my debut book *The Corridor That Lies Between Greatness And Insanity*, a practical book on how to deal with struggle God's way. You'll find there also that God gives us visible signs, very intriguing things to say the least.

Anyhow, I've compiled a myriad of stories that deal with the full spectrum of emergency calls – all of which are true. I could use fancy 10 codes, signal commands and confusing medical jargon, but that would make for a dizzy read. Some terminology simply cannot be avoided to tell the tales the way they should be told. But I have explanations of these terms and such, when used, so that the waters don't get too muddy for you. My desire for you in regards to these tales is to be entertained, educated and enlightened (enlightened by the Scripture). A life is important, yes, but your soul is *eternal*— have your heart in the right place and your priorities in line, if you catch my drift. We're all going to expire and no one's making it out of here alive.

We paramedics are present for the beginning of life as well as the devastating last breaths someone takes before crossing over to "the other side". Oh, and let's not forget all of the filth, vomit, blood, scum, sputum and sickness that surfaces in between life and death. Enjoy the true tales I've left for your liking and if you don't take away anything but this, don't forget it: love your neighbor as yourself. In other words, love your neighbor *like* you love yourself. Hold your loved ones just a little bit tighter and a little bit longer. Savor the moments you have while opposing decisions of regret. Be safe out there and God Bless you.

Paramedic Pointer» Don't waste your time with presumptuous-ness and pride; vanity is meaningless. In due time, we will all return to dust, from which we came from. If you don't believe me, visit a nursing home or a hospice.

Billions of runners around the globe racing to the finish, have they lived a fulfilled life, or did life wastefully diminish?

The gunshot of birth marks the beginning of the dash; an annual birthday bell rings, marking each contestant's lap.

Vanity infects the youthful with haughty eyes upon their face; aging is only fiction, they say, "I am in first place!"

But the street clinician knows from traveling place to place, that the younger in age only means further behind within the race.

All must finish — no matter the rate or pace. Whether in tragedy or triumph, death inevitably awaits.

Many lost ones look above, in search of a full moon, to sway into the night and drink until they swoon.

But truth is found in the morning star, in time these words will prove; there is only one way to an eternal win, a myriad to lose.

Understanding breeds objectivity, know this and one shall exploit: all are in the same race, the only contrast is one's checkpoint.

Lorenzo Hogans II

*The Lord is good, a strong hold in the day of trouble; and he knoweth them that trust in him **Nahum 1:7***

#1

Suffocation Before My Eyes

Paramedic Pointer» *Without oxygen, irreversible damage starts to occur to the brain within 4 to 6 minutes.*

"Is anybody answering the door?" I asked Larry, one of the firemen responding to a call tagged as a *medical alert*. A medical alert merely means that someone's medical necklace was activated. The elderly wear this so that all they have to do is press a button in case of emergency. "All the doors seem to be locked. I've tried the front door, the side door and even the garage door," Larry proclaimed. My partner Jeff and I double checked each door behind him for our own satisfaction. Sure enough, everything was locked. No lights were on either; at least it appeared that way when looking through the windows. But the curtains were closed, so it wasn't a very dependable gauge.

Medical alert tags are often activated by mistake, this possibility was apparent in each of our minds. "Maybe it was an accidental activation," Jeff said. "No one appears to be at this address." We stood in the front lawn of the residence looking for the best way to gain access. "I'd hate to break a window or door; whenever I can avoid damage, I do," Larry stated. Larry's partner, Lou, chimed in, "We gotta do what we gotta do… there could be somebody in there."

Standing just outside the front door, we knocked viciously, calling out for an audible answer from inside the house. No answer came. Sometimes there is a fallen patient in the rear of the house who simply cannot get up, and even if they heard our yells, could not yell loud enough to be heard from their location inside the house. "I'll go around the back, I think I saw a screened in patio," Larry reasoned. Moments later, Larry came from the backyard sprinting full speed. Before this call, I hadn't seen Larry race that fast for anything; not even walk fast. He was generally a slow mover. "Someone back there?" I asked in a frantic fluster. Larry didn't even respond to my question, he just kept running out to his fire truck as if he'd seen an alligator. By the time Jeff and I grabbed our stretcher to head towards the rear of the house, Larry was already sprinting passed us again, going in the same direction. This time, he had a screwdriver in his hands.

"She's back here! She's back here! We gotta get in!" he yelled.

There was a screened in patio with an in-ground pool inside. Luckily, the screen door was unlocked; we didn't even have to tear through it. What I saw next made my adrenaline go through the roof. Looking through the sliding glass door separating the living room from the pool deck, I saw an old woman holding her throat. She was trying her best to catch her breath, turning bluer by the second. She was sweating profusely; an extreme sense of impending doom was upon her— and all of my crew as well. Larry and the other fireman were having trouble prying the sliding glass door off of its tracks, so Jeff and I had to wait until they popped it off of its groove. It was gut-wrenching. We stood there watching an elderly woman *suffocate* right before our eyes.

"I'm not gonna sit here and watch her suffocate in front of me," I thought to myself. I backed up as far as I could, preparing to hurl myself through the glass door. My heels were on the edge of the pool. Just as my heels began to lift, in motion for a full-fledged Sprint, Larry announced, "I got it!"

My heart sank.

My focus immediately turned towards our medical bags— primarily the *oxygen* bag. We made it inside just in the nick of time. I'll never forget the look our patient gave me. It was a look of, "Thank God." Supplying her with oxygen, her color slowly began to return. Her lungs were filled with fluid; she had a cardiac condition called *CHF* (congestive heart failure). It's where fluid backs up into the lungs from the heart being overworked. We blasted her with oxygen to assert a positive improvement in her oxygen readings. She would be okay. We monitored her on the way to the hospital, ready for any further interventions necessary. She was elated to be alive and we felt the same. It was truly a close call— as close as it has ever been.

For his anger endureth but a moment;in his favour is life:weeping may endure for a night but joy come in the morning.
Psalm 30:5

#2

Red Wine Vomit

Paramedic Pointer *» The medical term for vomit is emesis. Coffee ground emesis is a classic sign of upper gastrointestinal bleeding. Bright red emesis is an indicator of a lower gastrointestinal bleed.*

Night time traffic is virtually none at all after midnight. When responding to a call, we rarely have to use the obnoxious air horn simply because there are no vehicles on the road. At about 2:30 AM dispatch notified us that someone called for a person who had altered mental status. With no traffic backup to slow us down, our response time was probably about half of what it usually is. Pulling up to a house with an outside porch light on, we stopped here although we could not make out the faded numbers on the residence. From responding to calls for years, my partner and I were both aware that some patients would leave an outside light on during the nighttime hours to make their house easily stand out. Even though this meant the right house more often than not, I briskly jogged up to the front door to confirm that the numbers matched our address given by dispatch. There was no point in pulling our cot all the way to the front door only to be greeted by some angry person who is disgruntled about us showing up without request (which happens every once in a while). I signaled to Jeff that we were in the right location. There was just enough room to squeeze our stretcher in between the left side of the three cars lined up in the driveway and the tall bushes that bordered the front lawn. We proceeded to the light in the screened in porch which had a pool table in it. A man with no shirt on, blue jeans and a shark tooth necklace greeted us in an anxious manner. Breathing heavily, he pointed down the hallway, followed by "she's down that way… She's thrown up about five times already… she's sick". Advancing down the hall, we entered a filthy room that not only smelled of vomit, but lemony fresh urine as well. On the bed laid our patient, who was wearing a torn silk nightgown. Her bed had no sheets on it for some reason. Maybe it was because she had already vomited and removed them. Nonetheless the mattress was filled with reddish colored pools of grainy barf. This woman was pale and obtunded (lights were on but no one was home). She was lying on the bed as if she was attempting to make snow angels, although in this case they would have been referred to as "vomit angels". She stared at the ceiling while lying on her back, mouth open as if she was witnessing something far-fetched. We sat her upright on the edge of the bed. Jeff and I positioned ourselves on each side of her, grasping her arms to help her attempt to walk a few steps to a chair a few feet away. "You will have to help her!" shouted the woman's boyfriend. He chose an interesting time to yell this, as we were already in motion towards the chair we were moving her to. The boyfriend paced back and forth frantically shaking his head. "I don't know what I'm going to do! I'm getting ready to lose it if you all don't do something!" A huge dog came running around the corner at this point and jumped on him, appearing to want to play. Thank goodness for the dog distracting him, I had never been happier to see a dog on scene of a 911 call—the dog served as a much-needed deterrent of this soon-to-be hostile man. "Can you lock the dog up for us sir? We can't have your pet getting in the way". He took the dog to some back room down the hall and around the corner. Sitting the woman down, Jeff grabbed our laptop to begin documenting while I reached for wires to place on the woman from our cardiac monitor. I heard a small noise that sounded like a belch coming from the patient. When I looked back (my back was turned) to glance at her there was a continuous flow of dark red vomit tumbling out of her mouth like a waterfall. Emesis bags (vomit bags) were kept on hand in our monitor for this very reason. I snatched one and caught what I could of her vomit. Her boyfriend came back at this point, and with a calmer demeanor, fortunately. "She drank an entire bottle of red wine tonight", he said. Aha, there was the culprit. She was drunk! She had consumed so much red wine to the point that she was plastered and her body rejected it! After the episode of waterfall-like vomit, she began to slur short phrases that made little to no sense. Since her nightgown was now submerged in throwup, we asked her boyfriend if he could find us another nightdress to slip her into. He immediately began filing through her dresser on a keen mission to be a help to us. "She's got so many clothes, I can't seem to find a nightgown", he said in a discouraging tone. "Awww... You don't have to do that, Joe..." She managed to slur. All of a sudden the room got quiet. No longer was the boyfriend shuffling through her wardrobe with a determined look on his face. Something is wrong, I thought to myself. When I glanced over at the female patient's boyfriend, who was still standing at the dresser, I saw the life in his entire body escape into thin air. He dropped his head, as well as his arms in a way that spelled dismay. Next, he gathered a look of both betrayal and fury as he asked, "JOE...? WHO'S JOE...? I'M NOT JOE!!" Oh no, not right now, I thought, drama is the last thing we need right now. Jeff and I began to expedite getting her onto the cot. Her vomit-tinged hair slapped me in the cheek. We rolled her out of the house as fast as we could. Her boyfriend did not turn violent luckily, retaining his anger with bawled fists, aggravated paces back and forth and cherry-red ears that looked as if they were going to shoot out fire. Upon loading the patient into the truck, I administered a drug called Zofran, which helps the patient to stop vomiting. Also, I hung a bag of fluids to replenish what fluids she had already lost from barfing. She was going to be okay. Rolling down the freeway en route to the ER, I had only feelings of gratitude that this call was not blown completely out of control with the drama that could have given us all a different outcome.

Though he fall, he shall not be utterly cast down: for the Lord upholdeth him with his hand. **Psalm 37:24**

#3

Entry Wound, Exit Wound

Paramedic Pointer» *Entry wounds from gunshots are typically smaller than the exit wound.*

In zone 16, a zone where crime is expected, gunshots echoed inside the walls of the ghetto apartment complex. A shooting had taken place that left only one gang member visible and it was because he was wounded, leaving him left behind when the rest of the posse "ran for the hills" so to speak. Abruptly stopping just steps away from the three police cars brought into focus the yellow caution tape that cordoned off the crime scene. Peering over near a wooden fence revealed a black male sitting in a chair with his head down, accompanied by a policeman and two firemen who were already on scene. Our pre-arrival notes showed that the patient had a gunshot wound; so we knew that time was of the essence. In dealing with trauma calls, loss of blood can greatly affect patient outcomes, so interventions must be swift. I grabbed the trauma kit, placing it on the cot and rushed towards our wounded patient. A blood soaked towel was wrapped around the young black man's left foot. He grimaced in pain, his head sweating bullets down his face—he was in great distress. I slowly unwrapped his left foot to examine his wound. On the left side of his left foot was where the bullet appeared to have entered; the right side of his left foot was where it exited. In contrasting an entry wound versus an exit wound, entry wounds are smaller than exit wounds. I left his foot exposed as I dropped the blood soaked towel to grab some gauze and cling (cotton bandaging material) to give his foot a fresh dressing (dressing is simply the term we use when wrapping a wound). My hope was that he didn't look at the gunshot holes as I grabbed the supplies out of the trauma bag. The gaping holes in his foot were absolutely gruesome. Every layer of his flesh was visible, not a site for the squeamish. "What is your name, sir"? I asked. "Aaahhh…!!… Kevin!! He replied. He explained of how a gang rivalry led to a drive-by shooting from another crew against his crew. "We recognized the car we all knew to mean trouble rolling down its window and the next thing I knew, gunshots fired at us", Kevin said. "I was just a few feet away before I could turn the corner when I got hit in the foot…I was running fast", he said between heavy breaths. "I had to pull together all the will I had to hop with my other foot around the corner", Kevin said while shaking his head in disbelief. "Let's get you fixed up… We've already got your foot wrapped and now we're going to give you some morphine to alleviate the pain", I told him with reassurance. "Please, PLEASE hurry! I can't take it anymore!" Kevin yelled in discomfort. His vital signs were normal, giving me the go ahead to proceed in morphine administration. Morphine makes quite a few people nauseous so I preceded the morphine with the drug Zofran to prevent him from vomiting.

In order to track whether or not a person's pain is subsiding or not, we use a pain scale. We simply ask the patient how bad his or her pain is on a scale of 1 to 10, 10 being the worst pain you've ever felt in your life. This pain scale allows us to record trends, trends meaning continuous documentation throughout a call to let us paramedics know if our patient is declining or stabilizing. So five minutes after the first dosage was pushed, Kevin's pain was still very high. His pain scale had moved down only one point, a 9 out of 10. It was time for a second dose. "Could you hurry up with the meds, this pain is just too much! Kevin pleaded. Pushing the second dose of morphine, I then reevaluated Kevin's vital signs and they were looking better. When checking his pain scale again, it had only moved down one more point, an 8 out of 10. More powerful than morphine is another narcotic called Dilaudid, this was to be given next. Kevin's pain was immense – holes in your foot the size of quarters will create that kind of pain. The Dilaudid lowered his pain down to a 6 out of 10, which appeared to be tolerable. Kevin's torso was submerged in tattoos that told many stories without words. His arms were covered in sleeve tattoos that reflected gang-related symbols and insignias. Kevin's current predicament had clearly been a side effect of his lifestyle. "I can't live like this anymore", Kevin said with his face buried in his hands. "I've got a daughter who needs me; I'm lucky that it was only my foot", he said in a sentimental tone. "I won't argue with you there", I replied in agreement. "I'm only 28 years old, I can't die yet", he said as if his life flashed before him in an instant. "It's never too late to change your lifestyle", I replied. Unloading Kevin out of the ambulance, we entered the busy ER to drop him off with a nurse. He was to receive an x-ray and talk with the Doc soon. Before I turned the corner I popped my head back through the privacy curtains and reminded him that it wasn't too late to change his lifestyle. Kevin replied "You're right, thanks a lot for everything". "You're welcome", I said, sealing our parting of ways with a handshake.

Thou, which hast showed me great troubles and sore troubles, shalt quicken me again, and shalt bring me up again from the depths of the earth. **Psalm 71:20**

#4

A Bullet in the Liver Will Make You Quiver

Paramedic Pointer» *Located in the upper right quadrant of your abdomen, the liver's primary functions is the filtering of blood and the production of bile, which helps carry away waste and break down fats.*

Jeff was taking a shower. I was changing into my jumpsuit that had reflectors on it for nighttime visual clarity. It was approximately 10:45 PM, Jeff and I had run our tails off all day long. My *hamburger helper* was almost done, I hoped desperately to be able to devour it because while the call volume was high, the contents in my stomach were low. I managed to slurp half of my meal down when the station bells rang for another call. Clasping my belt around my waist, which had my radio on it, I poked my head in Jeff's restroom to shout, "We've got a call! It's time to roll!" Jeff came hopping around the corner fumbling with his socks as he attempted to slide them over his wet feet. "What did the call come in as?" Jeff asked me in a hurried voice while jostling his feet into his boots. "A gunshot wound", I answered.

Swerving through traffic like a serpentine, we found ourselves in a street that looked like they were having a block party. Unfortunately, this was not the case; however, there were about six cop cars along this neighborhood street. And on top of that, what seemed to be the entire neighborhood was gathered around the patient, staring at him with curiosity. Picture the kind of crowd a packed concert brings. If you've ever been to a packed concert or similar scenario where you have to "get skinny" or turn sideways to slip passed people due to the congestion, then compare that with this scenario. People were bunched up together as if this were some kind of exhibit to behold. But this wasn't going to work at all; Jeff and I needed to get to the core of this congestion immediately. "Everyone back up and let us through!" We shouted with authority. Realizing that help was here, the neighborhood spectators began to make a pathway for Jeff and me to come through. Once we reached the center of the crowd, we saw a young black male on his back in nothing but *Batman* boxers. He had dreads that looked to be 8 to 10 inches long; the wounded patient was rocking side to side on, holding his abdomen. His face was turned upward; his straining accompanied his scrunched up facial expressions. Grunting every few seconds, the patient managed to say, "they shot me man!" Every movement he made strongly suggested that this patient was in a great deal of pain. He was sweating profusely, he was guarding (holding) his abdomen and grunted in painful spurts… But we didn't see a gunshot wound anywhere. "Where did you get shot?" I asked the man. He opened his eyes wide and lifted his head off of the driveway concrete, opening his mouth to say something but no words came out. He pushed out a painful sigh as his head lowered slowly back down to the cement. Kneeling down next to him, I rapidly assessed his anterior. I found no culprit for a gunshot wound. Jeff and I quickly rolled the patient onto his right side so that we could evaluate his posterior…there it was. On the young black man's lower back was the bullet hole. I felt around the bullet hole with a gloved hand to feel for the actual bullet. We knew that it was inside his body because there was only one bullet hole present, there was no exit wound.

We placed the patient onto our stretcher and asked him his name as we buckled him in. "Manny", he whispered due to the pain. By this time, the large crowd of spectators had spread out a lot more, making getting to our rig a lot more easy than snaking through a clump of people like we did when we first arrived on scene. I lifted the stretcher into the ambulance and locked it in place. In checking his vital signs, (blood pressure, heart rate, breathing rate, etc.) Manny's blood pressure was a bit low. With Manny having been shot, it was almost inevitably due to an internal bleed. I started an IV in Manny's left arm so that we could deliver some fluids into his body, intending to raise his blood pressure. Because for those of you who don't know, if your blood pressure tanks (goes to zero or in other words, becomes nonexistent) then you are clinically dead. Before you die however, there is a stage of low blood pressure referred to as "shock". Shock is undesirable as well. We were able to raise Manny's blood pressure, allowing us to then give pain medication. Morphine helped the pain to subside until we got to the ER. "How are you feeling Manny?" I asked as I opened the rear ambulance doors. "A lot better but it still hurts," he responded. Since Manny was deemed as what we refer to as a "trauma alert", we transported him with lights and sirens on, which is typical done *on the way to* the patient. So we arrived very quickly at the ER and the trauma team was gowned down and gloved up. The Doc in the trauma room asked for the run down on Manny and we proceeded to give him the scoop. "How much medication did you administer?" The Doc asked. "4 mg of morphine", I replied. "Bring in the x-ray!" The doctor ordered. Jeff and I moved Manny over to the hospital bed to be further evaluated by the trauma team. Just a few minutes after snapping a few shots of Manny's torso, it was declared that the bullet pierced Manny's liver. I looked over and saw Manny beginning to twitch and shake. Nurses and ER medics expedited their patient care as soon as the x-ray machine was removed. Manny would soon be on his way to receive surgical care for the removal of that bullet. "What a night", Jeff turned and said to me. "No doubt about that", I replied, reloading our supplies for the next round.

Though I walk in the midst of trouble, thou wilt revive me: thou shalt stretch forth thine hand against the wrath of mine enemies, and thy right hand shall save me. **Psalm 138:7**

#5

Brawl On The Beach

Paramedic Pointer» *It isn't uncommon for assaults to result in a person acquiring a hematoma or a contusion. A contusion is a "bruise" and a hematoma is a "lump on the head" caused by the pooling of blood below skin.*

Memorial Day weekend brought about a multitude of people out to Holmes Beach, Florida, the location my partner and I were assigned to on this particular shift. Our dispatcher advised us to use caution by staging a block or two from the call. Our assignment was to respond to an assault on the beach that was phoned in by a bystander. Staging until the police department arrives on a violent scene is a normal precautionary measure to take because weapons, wild behavior and other safety hazards are best dealt with by police.

"PD (Police Department) is now on scene, you may proceed to the scene at your discretion", dispatch told us. "Here we go", Jeff said as he let out a big breath and pressed the gas pedal. We rolled up slowly into a beach parking lot where men and women were scrambling in a frenzy. I slipped a set of gloves on. "Just watch yourself", Jeff warned me. I nodded in acknowledgment to his word of caution and made my way to the first person I saw. A man was standing in the middle of the lot, staring off into the distance with a baffled look on his face. "What happened", I candidly asked the man. He seemed to have been the only individual who wasn't running around like a chicken with his head cut off. "They were just here…" He said, maintaining a look of awe. "Who was just here? Who's *they*?" I asked. "A gang of about 30 people… They had guns and blades…" He said fizzling out at the last few words, making them just barely audible. "But what exactly happened? Did they attack anyone?" I questioned. "My buddies and I were coming back in from the water on our jet skis where the boats offload into the water. There was an all-black suburban trying to offload a boat into the water but realized we were in the way. The driver got out and asked us what we were doing in an aggravated manner and I told him we were moving. I also told him that my friends and I weren't looking for any trouble and he just got back in his suburban without saying anything. I figured everything was cool but the next thing I know, five more black suburban SUVs showed up and like 30 guys jumped out and ganged up on my buddies and I. It was like 30 versus five. I personally keep a knife on me at all times, but there was so many of them that there was no time to even reach for it while I was getting kicked in my head", he explained. Apparently looking for someone, he turned to face the opposite direction with his chin held high and his eyes squinted. Until now I had only seen his left side. His right side now in view, startled me because his entire ear was hanging from his head. There was literally a thin strip of flesh keeping his ear from falling to the ground. What a bloody mess it was, and shocking to say the least. He had not even mentioned his ear being sliced almost completely off thus far. So I prompted him with an interruption, "how did that happen to your ear?!" He turned and looked at me slowly with a look of pure fear in his eyes, "two guys attacked me; once I fell to the ground, one of the guys held my face down against the concrete with his boot while the other one took a knife out and sliced my ear almost all the way off". Jeff rushed over to let me know that the four other men involved just had bruises and scrapes. He also made it clear that the big frenzy was scared families running to their cars, collecting their children on the way. "Let's get you into the truck", I told the Caucasian male. "I don't think I want to go to the hospital sir", he replied. "Your ear is practically about to fall off, let's get inside the truck and stop the bleeding if anything", I suggested. He sat on the bench seat inside the ambulance and allowed us to evaluate his ear further. We took his vital signs as well as double checked his body to see if he had any other injuries. He ended up receiving a circumferential wrap around his head to hold his ear up from dangling, which also helped stop the bleeding at the same time. "You will definitely need to be seen at a hospital", I told him. "I understand. I will. But I'm going to have my wife take me up to the hospital in our car". The bleeding was managed with the circumferential dressing around his head. No other injuries were to be found so I had him sign a 'refusal of transport' form on my laptop. A handful of knocks were heard coming from the rear ambulance doors. Letting our patient out, one of the men involved in the parking lot brawl stood there holding his ribs on his right side. "The pain is so bad that I barely even want to take a breath because it makes the pain intolerable", the now second patient explained. He was not strong enough to step up onto the ambulance. I unloaded the cot, lowered it and had him take a seat on it so that we could load him into the truck without him having to exert himself at all. "I thought I was going to be just fine a few moments ago but I guess my adrenaline rush wore off", he sighed. "I'm Lorenzo and this is my partner Jeff. What's your name?" "Todd", he answered. "So what happened to you Todd? Is the only pain you feel in your right rib area"? "Three or four guys ganged up on me, threw me to the floor and started punching me, nonstop, in my side", Todd answered.

I took the shears off of the hook on the ambulance interior wall and snipped off his shirt. Trauma shears are emergency scissors that we use in the field to cut off clothing in order to assess an injury site. His ribs felt like they were cracked. I felt his left ribs to compare both sides. Feeling the opposite side confirmed the deformity. In the prehospital setting, there are no x-ray machines to tell whether or not a bone is broken. Therefore, unless it is blatantly obvious, we paramedics cannot say for sure if a bone is fractured. In many situations, yes—but not all. "What is your pain on a scale of 1 to 10, 10 being the worst pain you've ever felt in your entire life"? I asked Todd. "Umm…" Todd started, attempting to make his reply heard through pain. "And 8 out of 10", Todd said. Todd was administered pain meds to cope with his rib pain on the way to the hospital ER. An x-ray indeed confirmed that there were broken ribs on his right side. Todd would then need ample time to heal. Memorial Day, it is an American day to remember those who died in the military while in active service. Todd, however, now has an additional event to remember when it comes to this holiday.

Many are the afflictions of the righteous: but the Lord delivers him out of them all. **Psalm 34:19**

#6

Mike Tyson's Successor

Paramedic Pointer» *Blood vessels constrict when they get cold, which is why we administer ice packs to traumatic bruising. When veins are constricted it doesn't allow as much blood to pool in the immediate area under the skin. Constricted Veins = Less blood pooling = Less swelling.*

It's 2 AM. I'm sound asleep in my station bed. Emergency tones sounded off, alarming me to wake up out of a slumber so peaceful, it could have been compared to a sleep an infant gets when sung their favorite lullaby. Another assault. According to the call notes, there were two women involved in a physical confrontation. The police department had already made it on scene, so there wasn't any need for us to stage for safety reasons.

KNOCK-KNOCK-KNOCK… "Hello?! Paramedics! Anyone home?!" Three cop cars were in the residence driveway and the address definitely matched the address we were given so without further delay, I turned the doorknob slowly, taking my first step across the front door's threshold. Everything was trashed. Garbage was thrown all over the place, the chandelier was hanging unbalanced and I also noticed a broken vase. An altercation had taken place in this residence—and I could tell that it was a fiery one indeed because I could feel the "heat" from the fight lingering in the open space in a way. "HELLOOO!" Jeff yelled as we continued onward, deeper into the home. A voice from a back room suddenly became audible, "back here… we're back here"! Navigating through an obstacle course of a mess, Jeff and I both noticed small trails of blood ingrained in the carpet. Just around the corner was a bedroom where the police and one woman were exchanging words with one another. A second after Jeff and I entered the bedroom, a cop who was writing information down on his notepad turned towards us and exclaimed, "This young lady got into a fight with her girlfriend and it resulted in her ear being bitten off". "Must've been a nasty scuffle", I thought to myself while approaching the black woman. She looked to be in her mid-30s. She was crying with a paranoid look on her face, intermittently looking around as if someone was still after her. She had big, poofy hair that covered both of her ears. I stepped in and moved her hair back to expose both of her ears. Sure enough, her right ear was 75% gone. Only the top quarter was still attached. "What's your name miss"? I asked. "Christina," the woman replied, as she sunk her head into her cupped hands and broke down into tears. Christina quickly dried her eyes and regrouped in an earnest attempt to hold things together. "Can you do anything for my ear"? Christina inquired, eyes still watery. She looked as if she was a desperate patient in a hospital waiting to hear if she would live or die. And rightfully so, I suppose, no one wants to lose their ear. "They may be able to reattach it at the hospital Christina, but where is the ear"? I inquired. Blood slowly dripped from what was left of her right ear on to her shoulder as she pointed towards the kitchen and said, "It's in the freezer". We began to make our way to the freezer to examine her detached ear. "I placed it in a Ziploc bag and put it in the freezer to try and preserve it", Christina informed while walking with me.

Opening the freezer brought about an unexpected surprise. The detached ear was exactly how Christina described — in a plastic Ziploc bag. Only, to Jeff and I's surprise, it still had a very large hoop earring in it. I took it out of the freezer and held it up in the kitchen light. Christina's detached ear had shriveled down considerably. Christina asked, "So do you think they can reattach it for me at the hospital"? "Nope, unfortunately that ear is too shriveled up from necrosis (tissue death)", Jeff interjected. "Are you sure? I placed it on ice… That should have preserved it right"?? Christina pleaded in disappointment.

Jeff, who had been a bit restless at the time, shrugged his shoulders and said, "we'll just look at it, it's black as h…" Jeff paused and went mute before finishing his sentence. He looked at me as he abruptly held his tongue. Thank goodness he didn't let what we all know he was getting at come out of his mouth because our patient was an extremely dark African-American woman. Somehow I don't feel that had he finished his statement, it would have fared well with our patient — especially coming from a nerdy white guy. "So how did the fight evolve between you and your girlfriend"? I asked. "She got angry when I told her that I was moving to Winterhaven (approximately two hours from where she currently lived). My girlfriend started tearing up the house, threatened to bang up my car and that's when she jumped on me and bit my ear off", Christina explained in an overly timid voice. "Where's your girlfriend now, Christina"? I inquired. "She ran out of the house after she bit my ear off. But she did threaten to come back and trash my car", Christina said as she began to cry again. "Would you like to go to the hospital by ambulance or your personal vehicle"? I asked. "No I'm scared my ex is going to come wreck my car while I'm gone"! Christina cried out. "Well, allow us to double check everything inside the truck, okay"? I strongly suggested. Christina allowed Jeff and I to do so. She then decided that taking her own vehicle was how she would transport herself to the ER.

Ultimately it made no difference because with Christina being completely stable, there was nothing outside of "giving her a ride" that we could do for her. Even if her ear was re-attachable, we paramedics do not do stitches — it simply isn't in our scope of practice. Taking her own vehicle also provided a way back home for her, she had stated earlier that she had no one who could pick her up if transported by ambulance. Christina's outcome was unfortunate, yet her life will go on. Her actual eardrum was not tampered with or damaged so it's not as if losing the exterior cartilage removes her ability to hear.

"I'm reeeaaalllyy glad you didn't finish your comment, Jeff", I joked. Jeff laughed and said, "No doubt, I'm glad I caught myself too because that would NOT have been pretty"! He said as we drove back to the station in the still of the night.

For the Lord will not cast off forever: but though he caused grief, yet will he have compassion according to the multitude of his mercies. For He does not afflict willingly more grief the children of men. **Lamentations 3:31 – 33**

#7

Trailer Park BOGO

Paramedic Pointer» *Paramedics do not have x-ray machines on our trucks contrary to some beliefs. We can make inferences and solid assessments in addition to obvious dislocations and fractures, but no x-rays, which is the only way to be 100% sure of a broken bone.*

*S*ugarcreek Mobile Home Park consistently produces calls in one fashion or another. Midday, when the sun was at its highest, we were requested for "leg pain". Little did we know that we had been enrolled in a buy one get one deal (hence the story title). *Sugarcreek Mobile Home Park* was your average mobile home community. It wasn't trashy per se, just a small community of retired seniors taking it easy. "Leg pain" is a broad term which can mean anything from a sore leg due to pulling a muscle to having a mangled leg from a machinery incident. A man with a khaki colored camping hat greeted us at the door.

"Marty can't get out of his chair; he's in so much pain!" The senior citizen exclaimed. "What happened to him"? I asked. "He fractured his tibia and fibula (the bones in your leg below the knee) a few days ago. He's already been seen at a hospital for it. They even gave him pain meds, but the pain meds aren't working all that well". I turned to look at Marty in the living room to the right, propping himself up with a pair of crutches. Marty had a wife beater on and whitey tighties. On his lower right leg he had a bulky black cast on it to immobilize the movement of his lower leg. "So much for not being able to get out of the chair", I thought to myself. "I want to go to the hospital"! Marty announced. Looking at him with a bit of confusion, I questioned his intent, "Well Marty, what do you wish to get from visiting the hospital again when you've already been there a few days ago? They've even prescribed you pain meds and have given you a cast." Marty answered back with, "I can't stand the pain, even when I'm only sitting down in my recliner — and that's *with* the prescribed pain pills they've got me on!" "Okay", I responded. "We had better get you on some pants of some sort if we can manage to. What kind of medications are you on?" "The pain pills they gave me are called Dilaudid," Marty blurted out. "How about any meds you take on a regular basis?" I asked. "Well shucks, I've got a long list of them somewhere around here," Marty said. Marty's friend, the gentleman in the camping hat perked up and informed Jeff and I, "I know exactly where they are! I'll go back to Marty's bathroom and get them off of the sink!"

"Grab me a pair of pants too, will you Doug?" Marty added. "Sure, buddy," Doug answered. Doug came back with Marty's pants that already had a belt in them. "Ahhhh!" Marty moaned as I attempted to slide the pants up his legs. "Give me a second, give me a second!" Marty demanded. So there I was kneeling down in front of Marty until he finally got his bearings to give it another go. He lifted one leg at a time while still propping himself up on the crutches. Marty kept his eyes closed the entire time we put his pants on as a method of focus. He tried intently to avoid any further pain because according to him, it was excruciating. I instructed Marty to put most of his weight onto his uninjured leg once we managed to fasten the buckle on his belt. Beginning to turn and head for the door, Marty's friend, Doug, came walking around the corner with the bag of medications he went to retrieve from the bathroom counter. There was a step where the living room and hallway met making the living room about 4 to 6 inches higher up.

CLUNK-CLUNK!! Marty's friend, Doug, had tripped over the step, hitting his left shoulder on the wooden floor. "Jesus Christ!!" Doug blurted in sudden pain. "What are the odds?" I thought. I'm not sure who was more surprised out of Marty, Jeff and myself; we all stood there for a split second in disbelief. It was as if seeing Doug in pain alleviated Marty's pain because he had stopped moaning and watched his friend, Doug, wallow in discomfort — and he did so in complete silence — eyes glued. Jeff tended to Marty as I knelt down to a now-injured Doug, who rocked from side to side on his back like a turtle while holding his left shoulder. Amazingly, Doug turned over, using his right hand to help himself up from the ground to a standing position again. I offered a helping hand to Doug in getting back up and he snapped, "I got it, I got it — I'm a military sergeant!" Doug rejected a helping hand because he clearly was tough enough to deal with matters on his own — especially pain. I evaluated his shoulders. Doug's left shoulder was clearly dislocated. I compared his right shoulder to his left and they were like night and day.

When we paramedics can get the cot close enough to the patient in situations where the patient can't walk well, we utilize a *stair chair*. A stair chair is a chair on wheels that is much more compact and useful for navigating a patient through tight spaces. It also has tracks on the back for transitioning patients down stairs. Since Marty could not move very well — even with the crutches — Jeff ran and grabbed our stair chair so we could wheel Marty out from where he already was. Doug, however, was able to walk out to the ambulance. So Jeff and I had earned ourselves a deal. It was more than we expected, but things have a way of working out like that in the field of emergency medical services. You show up thinking you've got one patient, blink your eyes, and poof! You now have *two* patients to manage.

Marty sat in the stretcher once we put him in the truck, while Doug sat on the bench seat against the ambulance wall. The administration of pain meds in regards to Marty was bypassed since his pain was not "new pain" (pain from a new occurrence or injury), So I again asked Doug was he sure he could handle *his* pain. "Of course!" Doug announced. Shame on me for questioning his toughness and military merit, I should have known better. Keeping this in mind, we cruised on into the hospital property to relay our BOGO deal to a receiving nurse.

These things I have spoken unto you, that in me ye might have peace. In the world you shall have tribulation: but be of good cheer; I have overcome the world. **John 16:33**

#8

Elderly Couple In A Daze

Paramedic Pointer» *If you are injured and under the influence of alcohol, you must be alert and oriented enough to be able to refuse care. You must prove orientation to person, place, time and event (i.e. where you're at, what year it is, who the president is, etc.)*

An upper-class condominium establishment called *Perico Bay* generated an emergency call for my partner and I that required us to put on our detective hats unexpectedly. *Perico Bay* was a vast community filled with beautiful lakes, tennis courts and a clubhouse for its residents. It had a security hub at the entrance, where the guard operated the gigantic arm that lifted up and down to let cars through. The guard, who was asleep, almost fell out of his chair when Jeff briefly chirped the sirens next to the small security hub. His hat was pulled down over his eyes to block the sunlight, and as you may imagine, fell off of his head, prompting him to quickly snatch it off of the ground and press the button. He then gave us a friendly wave as we inched over a speed bump at about 5 miles per hour. Speed bumps are always a drag for big ambulances, there's so much weight behind ambulance cabs that you have to be very cautious when going over any sort of hump or pothole. So we took it easy over every speedbump in *Perico Bay* (which turned out to be about 10 when I counted).

Locating the correct place was not hard — it was the *gaining entry* that turned out to be the challenge. The residence sat in a cul-de-sac that had a wonderful pond behind it. It also had a steep driveway. I grasped the front door and attempted to turn it, but the door was evidently locked. I rapped on the wooden door a few times and no one came to the door. Jeff and I waited a couple seconds, followed by another attempt at getting someone to answer the door. Still no answer. Jeff walked around to the back side of the house. He came back around to the front and said, "I found a way in through their porch." We pushed our stretcher through their thick, grassy lawn and into a decent sized patio. Their grass looked to be *St. Augustine* grass and it was well kept—but it didn't do much for the small wheels our cot has when we wheeled it through the yard. Jeff eased the sliding glass door open and called out for a patient, "Paramedics are here! Where are you?" No answer. It's always an eerie feeling being in someone else's home and no one returns the call of your voice. We hadn't the slightest idea of where our patient or patients were. So we lurked around the home quietly, trying to find our caller or *callers*. In the kitchen there was no one. In the dining room was no one. All rooms seemed to have been empty except for one. One room we had not yet checked and that was the master bedroom.

Sitting upright against the side of his bed was an elderly man who looked to be in his 80s, staring off into the abyss with a puzzled look on his face. Just after discovering him, we heard a soft phrase of gibberish that was just barely audible. The soft spoken gibberish could have been compared to a three-year-old child's tone of voice. Connected to the master bedroom was a bathroom, where we entered to discover yet another patient. It was a woman who looked to be in her 80s as well. Both patients had expensive rings on their left ring fingers — we gathered that they must have been husband and wife.

"What's going on today?" I said with a raised voice. Neither patient answered with a coherent reply. The woman put together some sort of inter-galactic, spaced out response and the man just kept saying, "What...! What did you say?!" Even after we had asked him the question and our lips were no longer moving he continued asking us what we said in extremely loud yelps. His wife kept on babbling about who knows what as Jeff and I both stood in astonishment. Two patients were on the floor in a daze, so there had to be a culprit of some sort, we thought. Dementia is often a condition inherited with old age, but the continuous rambling each patient did led us to believe that something else may have been involved. "Where's my hearing aid?!" The old man shouted repeatedly.

I left the master bedroom instantly — but not for his hearing aids — they were not of any medical concern in terms of top priority. If I found his hearing aids then great, but I was searching for medications because it was a possibility that their prescribed meds would explain what was going on a bit better. No luck. No drawer in the entire kitchen had any meds in them. I happened to glance out onto the back porch and spotted two empty wine glasses. Next to the wine glasses was a tall *empty* bottle of wine. "They got wasted together," I concluded in my head. Chuckling to myself I thought, "It all makes sense now. This couple is in a daze because they are drunk!" "I found the culprit, Jeff!" I said while making my way back to the master bedroom. Holding the empty bottle up, I showed him the remnants of what had been an evening of intoxication. Jeff laughed. Smiling, he said, "You're never too old to get wasted." In the event that a person is not oriented to person, place, event and time, they are not eligible to refuse transport in my jurisdiction. There's also the risk of one of these patients having fallen and us just not knowing since we weren't there when it occurred. Because all we see upon arrival is where they are currently — which is on the ground. For these reasons, the elderly couple required transport according to our protocol. To our satisfaction, no injuries occurred upon assessing them and everything was going to be just dandy once the couple sobered up. And that in its self deserves a "cheers".

Better is little with the fear of the Lord than great treasure and trouble there with. **Proverbs 15:16**

#9

Where's Your Wallet?

Paramedic Pointer» *Heroin is extremely popular among the lower income demographic because it is so cheap. It is a cheap high and coincidentally, it is cheap to die. Heroin gets you so high that you end up unconscious and no longer breathing. Don't do drugs!*

Heroin is the drug of choice in Manatee County, Florida. A local report took statistics in the month of July 15' to find that there were 310 heroin overdoses during that month alone. That's an average of about 10 overdoses per day (related to heroin). Heroin users are running rampant in the county of Manatee — and if you ask me I would guess that Manatee County is the capital of the *world* in regards to heroin overdoses. See, you have to understand that Jeff and I run multiple heroin calls in pretty much every one of our 24 hour shifts. Our reaction to this particular call when it appears on our computer screen is no longer one of surprise. Rather, it's the look of someone who is washing their hands — no real enthusiasm on their face. What I'm getting at is that it has become *expected*.

I'm not sure exactly when it occurred, but heroin calls somehow went from occasional to a full-blown routine. Nonetheless, the fact that we are inundated with heroin users in Manatee County never takes away from the quality of care we provide. Often, Jeff and I just kind of look at each other and think, "Really? Another one?" But when it's show time, we perform efficiently and effectively — always. One man seeking a "high" generated an emergency when he ended up unconscious on the floor of his girlfriend's apartment. Heroin slows one's respirations down so much that eventually the person will literally stop breathing. Whether the user is looking to get high/commit suicide are aware of this fact is unbeknownst to me.

Our call was located on the second floor of an apartment complex called *Oak Mead*. Police were on scene due to the suspicion of illegal drug use. Jeff and I lugged all of our medical kits upstairs, preparing to evaluate our patient. "His name is Chad," one officer said when we walked into the apartment unit. "His girlfriend said that he definitely took heroin a little bit ago," the officer informed us.

Chad's body was lifeless. He laid there on the floor, unconscious, in a pool of sweat. His hair was soaked with sweat. His arms, legs, neck and face even had a shine to them, provided by the slippery wetness on his skin that reflected light. Chad's respirations were very slow. Dropping all of our medical bags, Jeff and I both dove in to intervene. Luckily, Chad had great veins to start an IV in, making it a quick process to start one in his right arm. Jeff drew up medication while an on scene firefighter assisted breaths for Chad, or in other words gave him artificial breaths manually by squeezing and oxygen filled *bag valve mask*. I've heard many people assume that paramedics do mouth-to-mouth, so I'd like to take the time briefly to discontinue that assumption. These days, we are sure to have a barrier device when breathing for someone. There's no sense in swapping spit with the patient. Or even worse — blood. Too many diseases. Too much bacteria involved. Our bag valve mask allows us to place a mask on patients and squeeze air into them — no mouth-to-mouth resuscitation necessary.

So about 15 seconds passed by until Jeff had the Narcan completely ready to be administered. He handed it to me and I pushed it immediately into Chad's vein. Narcan is a reversal drug for narcotics. Our truck stays fully supplied with boxes of Narcan so that we never run out. Narcan works by undoing the effects of narcotics by binding with cell receptors, waking the patient back up in usually less than a few minutes in my experience. And once again,

Narcan did the trick. About 10 seconds later, Chad began to regain consciousness. He slowly opened his eyes and looked at all of our faces from lying on his back. It has to be a peculiar experience being completely unconscious and waking up to a law enforcement unit, fire unit and paramedic unit.

When questioned about what he took, Chad did not deny as most do — interestingly enough. He knew what he took and had no problem fessing up to the truth. Chad had the attitude of, "what's done is done and if there are consequences then so be it." The presence of law officers typically scare people, causing them to deny illegal drug use out of fear of going to jail — but not Chad. He didn't care. Helping Chad up to his feet brought about a handful of other questions such as: "What time did you take it? Why did you take it? How much did you take? Did you take it to kill yourself?"

In the midst of the police playing 21 questions with Chad, a drama queen ran out from one of the side rooms in the apartment crying her eyes out. "Oh my gosh, Chad! I thought you were going to die! I'm so happy that you're not dead! I'm so happy that you're not dead!!" "I'll be fine," exclaimed Chad to his apparent girlfriend. "Is this your residence?" An officer asked Chad in a deep voice. "No… I live in Fort Myers, I came up to see Rachel, she used to live in Fort Myers too before she moved here," Chad explained. Jeff checked Chad's vital signs before we began to transition from the second-floor apartment unit to the ambulance. "Everything looks good right now!" Jeff announced. Chad had "come back to earth" and was worn out. He was very calm and quiet. Maybe it was the utter realization that he very well could have been dead right now instead of alive. Maybe it was the epiphany he may have had of needing to change his ways. Or maybe it was the thought of never seeing his girlfriend again. One policeman grabbed Chad's left arm in case Chad got dizzy and fell. I supported Chad's right side for the same reasons as we took the first few steps down the staircase. The stretcher awaited us at the bottom of the stairwell.

I was surprised that Rachel, Chad's girlfriend, had not said goodbye or some other sentiment — this was typical when a couple was on scene and one had to be transported. But then she proved me wrong. Out came Rachel, she raced so fast to the above safety railing that I thought she was going to flip over it, toppling over all of us walking down the stairwell. Out of breath,

Rachel leaned over the above railing and said, "Chad." Chad turned up and looked at her, still drowsy from the heroin… "Yeah, Rachel?" Here it came, the moment of true sentiment I had seen so many times before but never got old. Like your favorite romance movie that you could watch a gazillion times. She leaned over the rail so elegantly. So gracefully. So engaged. And then out of her mouth spilled the words we had all expected, or *didn't* expect, rather… "Chad…" Rachel said. "… Where's your wallet?"

As for me, this is my covenant with them, saith the Lord; my spirit that is upon thee, and my words which I have put in thy mouth, shall not depart out of thy mouth, nor out of the mouth of thy seed, nor out of the mouth of thy seed's seed, saith the Lord, from henceforth and forever. **Isaiah 59:21**

#10

You Should Have Let Me Die!

Paramedic Pointer» *There is a wide world of depressed individuals who resort to addictions via drugs, alcohol, sex and other activities. Don't hesitate to offer help to someone you see these extreme behaviors in. There are also numerous programs available to assist in dealing with these issues; all it takes is a phone call.*

An "unconscious person" is what the computer dispatch screen read, that was all we had to go by for a description. Understand that the reasoning behind being unconscious could be a multitude of things such as: faintings, drownings, trauma, asphyxiation, seizures, strokes, heart attacks, low blood sugar, shock, respiratory arrest, concussions, cardiac arrest, overdose, so on and so forth. It is essentially the paramedics' responsibility to gather what findings are available, once on scene, to properly treat the patient . 3:30 AM was the time this particular call fell into our laps.

It was a quiet night, a watchful owl sat in a tree above our station staring intently with its big yellow eyes. I always preferred night responses over day responses. Overall, it was much more peaceful to handle business in a non-congested, cooler environment opposed to a likely hot, crowded location during the day. Other than being woken up out of bed in the middle of the night, nighttime experiences are more enjoyable.

Station 16's bell was comparable to five daggers stabbing you in your eardrums. My agency wanted to make sure that you heard it when it was time for a response. So the tones pierced my ears, commanding me out from beneath my comforter and literally yoking my head off of my pillow. "Medic 16 en route," Jeff verbalized on the radio before taking off. Our ambulance lights lit up the road, we were like a giant disco ball rolling down the street. An update to our call notes told us that firefighters were already on scene providing assistive ventilations — which means that our unconscious patient could not breathe on their own any longer — the firefighters had to breathe *for* the patient. Swerving around our last corner was an abandoned gas station where we saw a few firemen on their knees assisting the patient. Jeff and I slipped our purple gloves on in preparation for action.

I unloaded our stretcher, which had our necessary equipment already resting on top of it. Had you timed Jeff and I's dash from the ambulance to the patient, it would have been comparable to a record of some sort. One thing we don't do is lollygag. And when a patient is unconscious, time is even *more* precious. A few seconds can make a big difference in the grand scheme of things. We stopped just a foot or two away from the patient, who was lying supine (on his or her back) being kept alive by the delivered breaths of the handy firefighters. Our stretcher has a locking mechanism, or "brake", on one of the wheels. I kicked the lever, activating the brake so that our stretcher would not roll away. "Do we have any history of what happened?" I quickly asked the firemen. "No, we've got nothing. All we know is that she was laying here just like this when we arrived. I urgently knelt down to feel for a pulse. The female patient was maintaining a pulse which meant her heart was beating, to my satisfaction. If you're not breathing well or at all, that's one thing. But if you're not breathing AND you don't have a pulse, that's a whole new ballgame, because in the latter case, we must immediately begin pounding on your chest. No, not ruthlessly assaulting you. *Pounding on your chest* is a reference to CPR. With no further delay, Jeff handed me a tourniquet to get an IV started while he lifted the female patient's eyelids to assess her pupils. "Her pupils are pin-point," Jeff informed me. Pinpoint pupils are a hallmark sign of narcotic use. It appeared that our female patient had most likely overdosed on heroin. But there wasn't any reason to guess at whether or not she used a narcotic because we were going to be giving her our very own narcotic antidote in about 10 more seconds. Narcan is the drug (medication) that I'm referring to, which actually could be called "Narcan't" because the narcotics in a person system *can't* suppress them any longer once receiving Narcan from us.

Applying the tourniquet exposed one decent vein — our female patient was what we paramedics refer to as a "tough stick" — a term we assign individuals who are hard to obtain an IV line on. I zeroed in on the one vein that looked like a legit recipient for my needle. I had one shot, potentially, so I needed to make this work. Time was ticking, our patient was in need. Beneath the skin I advanced the needle into her vein — at least that's what it looked like in the poorly lit parking lot of the abandoned gas station. Jeff had the *flush* patiently waiting for me in the palm of his completely opened hand. Had the flush not been in his hand, it would've looked like he wanted me to give him a "five". Oh, and the flush is a fluid-filled syringe that you hook up to the IV to see if the IV is good or not. If the fluid flows freely when pushed by the plunger, then the IV is a success. If not, then the area you entered will swell up which simply means you are not in the vein — try again.

When I put the flush to the test, it was flowing nicely! I had successfully succeeded in getting this hard stick in the dim lighting! Speaking of which, we are taught to handle low lit environments by way of "feeling the vein" instead of just looking for one. However, unconscious patients can sometimes be severely dehydrated or have low blood volume, leaving their veins very flat and undetectable to the touch. Administering *Narcan* caused the overdosed patient to wake up in about 20 seconds. Strangely enough, though, our female patient had a shocking attitude. Sometimes an overdosed patient will have an attitude because their "high" was just blown. After all, they did spend their money, whether a small or large amount, to achieve the high. Her comment suggested that this was *not* her reason for having an attitude.

She slapped both of her hands on the parking lot pavement while lying on her back and shouted, "Why didn't you just let me die!?" Everyone on scene quickly turned their heads and looked at her in baffled disbelief. "I don't have a reason to live for! You should have just let me die!!"

"Our job is to prevent people from dying," Jeff replied to her obscenity. "Well you shouldn't have shown up!" She violently snapped. Prehospital management isn't always glorifying. Not every patient is exactly happy to see you when you arrive to help them. It's unfortunate she felt that way but today was not her day to die, as much as she may have desired it to be.

He that loveth his brother abideth in the light, and there is none occasion of stumbling in him. **1 John 2:10**

#11

A Mirroring Effect

Paramedic Pointer» *For crying out loud, wear your seatbelt! One fluid motion of swinging your hand across your body into the buckle gets the job done, it's just that simple! Besides, you don't want to get a ticket from the police. Kill two birds with one stone, your safety and the safety of your wallet!*

My first call ever was as a 20-year-old who was both excited and scared half to death. The night prior to my first shift in my field internship portion of school, I may have only gotten about four hours of sleep. I know — what was I thinking, right? Excitement never allowed me to sleep much before an actual event. Anticipation built up my adrenaline to where my eyelids could not stay shut for long. The shift start time was 0430. My first stop on the way there was McDonald's, filling my empty stomach took priority over everything. I woke up that morning at about 0300. I needed enough time to get dressed, eat and travel to the EMS headquarters because the headquarters was about an hour away from my house.

Introducing myself to my preceptor with an extended right hand, she shook it firmly like a man and said, "Welcome to EMS, I'm Tabitha." Tabitha was short and stocky. I almost offered her my face shaver to get rid of the stubble on her chin. "First, we check out the ambulance to make sure all of our equipment and medications are there," she began. "You never know if the previous shift has fully restocked the truck's inventory or not," she continued. "The last thing we want to do is show up to a call and not have something that we need," Tabitha stated. Tabitha and I checked everything in the ambulance from top to bottom — including checking each and every one of the drugs for expiration dates. About 25 minutes following our tedious inventory review, we received a call for a traffic incident. A septic truck collided with a Chevy Cavalier. My heart rate went up — I could easily tell by the way my heart felt like it was beating out of my chest. Had there not been flesh on my chest to prevent it, my heart would have literally jumped out. Searching for my reflective vest for a few moments, a bit of relief came to me when I spotted it under the captain's chair — it must have fallen and slid under there by accident.

Next, I frantically placed my gloves on both hands. As far as the reflective vest goes, it's always a "must" when it comes to traffic incidents. Drivers aren't always paying attention, so they need all the help they can get to see you — reflective vests serve that purpose. So my first time riding down the street in an ambulance I was facing backwards (due to sitting in the back of the ambulance) bouncing up and down and holding on for dear life to the hand rail as we whipped around corners with screaming sirens blasting. Any "waking up" to do was done in a very short amount of time during this initial response.

The ambulance came to a halt on what had to be a four-lane road. Out the back of the ambulance I peered, nervous of what was to come next. There was a 96' Chevy Cavalier, which looked to be squashed into a paper ball, and a gigantic septic truck that had moderate front end damage. Two responders flung the rear ambulance doors open and I jumped out, ready to help where I could. "The firefighters are extricating the patient out of the vehicle; it should be a few minutes!" Tabitha yelled over the noisy scene commotion. I watched from just a few yards away — the large tools at work — slicing and separating heavy metal to free our patient.

Then, what appeared to be a mangled human was snatched out of the driver's seat and laid on the stretcher. Movements were superfast in getting the patient over to the ambulance. Two firefighter/paramedics lifted the young woman into the truck; I immediately dashed to the side ambulance store and jumped in to prepare for treatment. A bald firefighter/paramedic looked at me intensely following the slamming of the rear ambulance doors… "You! Start CPR!" He directed me. Locking my elbows, I began pumping on the young girl's chest. Blood spewed out of her mouth like a geyser! Each compression forced another splash of bright red blood out of her mouth. Looking at her reminded me of a zombie. She was mangled, all sorts of different colors and dead—to be exact. "This woman has suffered major trauma! She's 20 years old! She was T-boned by a septic truck!" The delegating fire medic informed everyone. There were a total of five people cramped in the back of the ambulance, all of who were attempting to intervene with a treatment of some sort.

Irony, in the sense that our patient was 20 years old, the same age as me at the time, struck me in an eerie way. Compressing her chest with as much quality as possible, I thought about how this woman had suffered a tragic misfortune. But why her? Why not me? Or why not any other 20-year-old for that matter? The hard statistics reveal that everyone is likely to be involved in at least one vehicle incident in their life, whether it's minor or catastrophically major. Further, humans are not perfect, leaving room for mistakes to introduce themselves in costly ways. Tabitha's partner successfully performed a process called intubation (where a tube is placed in your windpipe) so that we could breathe for the patient. Our patient had no pulse, however, so we had to deliver a few rounds of electricity to our female victim. No luck. 20 minutes or so of resuscitation could not revive her. When we got to the hospital, we officially pronounced her dead, followed by a doctor's confirmation shortly thereafter. "What a terrible outcome for my very first call," I thought. But I soon learned that the old phrase *you win some you lose some* also applied to the world of EMS. It's tough to accept as a paramedic, but the truth remains — you can't save everyone. The aroma of her blood had been lingering throughout the call, managing to settle inside my nostrils. I am, by no means, squeamish towards grotesque things, but the ongoing scent of blood can make a person nauseous. This is exactly what happened to me. I found myself exiting the ER as fast as I could to get some fresh air in the parking lot. Bending over in a grassy area,

I prepared to hurl — nothing came. False alarm. The fresh air must've helped because I was certain that my bacon, egg and cheese mcgriddle was going to resurface. A tall, dark security guard who could tell what I was going through, walked by, just as I stood back upright and said, "Ha… welcome to EMS," in a deep, humored voice.

*A new commandment I give unto you, that ye love one another;
as I have loved you, that ye also love one another. By this shall all
men know that ye are my disciples, if ye have love one to another.*
John 13:34 – 35

#12

Have You Seen My Friend?

Paramedic Pointer» Dementia is more than just memory
loss – most people associate dementia with memory loss, but the
condition affects people in a wide variety of ways. That might
include changes in behaviour, confusion and disorientation,
delusions and hallucinations, difficulty communicating, problems
judging speeds and distances and even cravings for particular
foods. Everyone's experience of dementia is different.

Clarence Smith was strong. When I say strong, I mean abnormally strong —
especially for a 74-year-old man. Clarence stayed in a nursing home. He
sat in a wheelchair because he was not able to walk. However, Clarence "stood"
so to speak, about 6'4" tall. He weighed approximately 260 pounds. His hands
could completely encompass an average sized hand, but you probably wouldn't
want to test it out with Clarence because when he latched onto something, it
was with a death grip. And good luck trying to pry his hand open, overpower-
ing him simply isn't going to happen. You need to sweet talk him or redirect his
focus somehow in order to succeed in escaping his death grip.

"Clarence has been increasingly aggressive today for some reason," one
of the nursing home aides stated. "He had fallen out of his wheelchair this

morning and we think he might have bumped his head, but no one witnessed his fall," the aide included. "He slapped the nurse today too," she added. If you were to take a glance at Clarence, you would've seen his usual grin. Clarence seemed as though he was easy-going — and he was — until someone got in his personal space. The first thing Clarence said to my partner Jeff and I was, "have you seen my friend?" He seemed to be worried about an acquaintance of his from the nursing home. Jeff and I figured that he just wanted to say goodbye before we transported him to the hospital; Clarence had a bump on his head from falling earlier that day. Lifting Clarence out of his wheelchair onto our stretcher took four people to be safe. Truthfully, we had all taken a gamble in doing so because Clarence could have assaulted any of us — and he was known to do so. Clarence had a gold tooth that shined bright each time he cracked a smile. He had a pleasant smile too, only it was accompanied often by a swift snatching of someone's wrist. Rolling Clarence down the hall of the nursing home required caution because he repeatedly tried to reach out and yoke a random nurse in passing. "Have y'all seen my buddy?" Clarence asked for a second time. "I've got to find him, I've been looking for him," he declared.

I was able to put the blood pressure cuff around his arm to my surprise. Clarence had stopped making sudden movements once inside the ambulance. The bump on his head was minimal with no bleeding. Assessing the rest of his body revealed no injuries. His questions about his friend continued, however. Clarence added some advice about how to find his friend finally. "Where did you last see him, Clarence?" I asked him. Clarence locked eyes with me, staring at me as if he could read my mind. He then opened his mouth slowly and began, "in order to find my friend you have to go deep inside to find the host." Wait. What? What on earth is Clarence talking about? Go deep inside to find the host? "Okay, are we even talking about a legit person at this point?" I wondered. "Let me feel your wrist, Clarence," I said while gently feeling for a pulse on his left wrist. It was normal — nothing to be concerned about as expected. Everything turned out to be completely stable for Clarence and so I took one last stab at finding out about this mysterious friend of his. I curiously asked, "What's your friend's name?" Clarence gazed at me for a moment with no words. "What's his name?" Clarence asked appearing to be startled. "Yes, his name — what's your friend's name?" I repeated. "I've got his bracelet he gave to me — his name is right here," Clarence explained as he pointed to his leather bracelet. I looked down to read the lettering on his bracelet to find that they spelled C-L-A-R-E-N-C-E S-M-I-T-H. Clarence had been trying to find himself all along.

For God so loved the world, that he gave his only begotten son, that whosoever believes in him should not perish, but have everlasting life. **John 3:16**

#13

The Burger King

Paramedic Pointer» *Schizophrenia affects 1% of the U.S. population. It is estimated that 50% of those people will have suffered the onset of schizophrenia as a result of a co-dependency on either alcohol, drugs or both.*

Oddly enough, we came across a patient who had all of us scratching our heads. All of us, meaning all of the police, firemen and paramedics who were on scene. From the "get-go" we knew generally what kind of patient we were dealing with, the location itself gave Jeff and I a big clue. The facility was named the *Manatee Glenns.* It was a psychiatric facility that housed patients dealing with substance abuse, suicidal thoughts/attempts and other citizens in the county who were generally just plain old coocoo. An 18-year-old girl tried to hang herself with her own shoe laces here. One gentleman thought he could dig through his solitary unit if he scratched enough at the walls. Another woman offered me to take the elevator to the top floor with her and jump off the building holding hands. I kid you not — she even expressed to me that she thought it would be romantic. Places like psychiatric facilities often gave me the creeps, especially ones that were kept up like one place that'll probably never scratch out of my memory bank called *Jacaranda Manor.* "What a ghastly name", I had thought, from the very first time hearing it — and even now. It's a shame but the name *Jacaranda Manor* was fitting. It looked like a haunted house from 1916. Inside smelled like rank urine. The walls had stains on them. And every room had some deformed or deranged looking individual inside that always seemed to be foaming at the mouth. Cries from multiple rooms made it sound like these people were being whipped and beaten. *Manatee Glenns* was more clean then *Jacaranda Manor*, however. Environmental cleanliness does wonders for a facility; I just wish it somehow improved the mental capacity of its residents.

Jeff and I were summoned for a man threatening to harm himself, he had been given a BA-52 — also known as a *Baker Act*. Baker acts are given to those who publicly make it known that they want to harm or even kill themselves. This was the reason he was at Manatee Glenns. Now, the reason paramedics (Jeff and I) were called is because he was behaving uncontrollably and needed medical clearance. The patient we had been summoned for was sitting in the corner, rocking lightly with his knees pressed against his chest. He hummed very softly, as if he was attempting to keep himself calm — like a mother's lullaby does for a baby. His eyes were wide like he had seen a ghost. His arms encircled his knees that were up against his chest, packaging himself as compact as he could. He gave off the vibe that he did not want to be noticed — remaining quiet and intentionally ignorant to our presence. "How about you stand up and talk to us Sir," I said initially. The patient didn't break his rhythm, continuing to keep his eyes wide open on the same spot on the lower wall 3 feet across from him. I'm not even sure if he blinked once since we had gotten in the room. "Sir, we're going to need you to cooperate with us so we can check you out," Jeff said after a few seconds passed. Still no break in his rocking motion. We were nonexistent to him. He remained detached, swaying back and forth on his bottom as if he were in a rocking chair. "Welp, better let him do his thing for a bit while we get his paperwork... No sense in disturbing him before it's time," Jeff suggested. A facility rep fetched our patient's paperwork and came back with a short stack of sheets in a manila folder. "Thank you," I said as the facility rep handed the paperwork over in a nervous manner. She was more than likely "shook up" by the patient's uncontrollable behavior from before we arrived. Psychiatric patients can get violent on a whim. Much like an on and off switch, bipolar patients, in particular, can go from cheerful to fearful in an instant; Or from glad to mad after a sneeze. The psychiatric tend to have bouts of extraordinary strength as well. Whether they are bipolar, schizophrenic, psychopathic, suicidal, hyper paranoid or extremely elevated in the category of anxiety, I've personally seen a 120 pound woman give five officers a run for their money. It's actually quite impressive to witness. "Okay, let's go ahead and get up Sir," Jeff suggested to the sitting patient. To my surprise, the man began to get up. Jeff extended a gloved hand to shake with in saying, "I'm Jeff, what's your name?"

"Don't yoouusss touch me!" The man snapped in an instant. He had the kind of ponytail that rests on the top of the head. The remaining hair hanging outside of his ponytail was shoulder length. It was dark brown — matching his scruffy beard and thick eyebrows. I saw that a pink scrunchy was what held his ponytail up. I began to be surprised about his color choice but quickly remembered that anything goes these days — especially with the mentally unstable. "I wrestle with the alligators in the swamps and kill raccoons with my bare hands! I come from the woods maaaannn..." He said in a tough guy kind of way. Jeff asked, "What's your name sir?" "… What?" The patient asked as if he was flummoxed. He stumbled backwards two steps, his hair swinging side to side and said, "…Uhh, my name?" "Yes, your name sir — what is your name?" Jeff asked again. "Uhh… Burger," the patient answered. "Really?" Jeff questioned. "Hmm, and what's your last name?" Jeff continued. "Uhh… King," the patient said. Jeff attempted to place his gloved hand on the patient's shoulder when it was evaded by our patient with a subtle deflection. "Don't yoouusss touch me! Meeess not feeling so good," the patient said as if he was a toddler. He got on the stretcher willingly, but once he sat down, he raised a finger quickly followed by another warning not to touch him. A fireman must have forgot his request once we got in the back of the ambulance because the fireman touched the patient on his shoulder, even though it was in a compassionate way. Burger King smacked the fireman in the face! "I told yoouusss not to touch me! Makes meeess upset!" The patient scolded. For some weird reason he always put an "S" on the end of his words. In slapping the fireman, Burger King only got more riled up with everyone trying to restrain him now. The four people in the back of the ambulance, including myself, were now forcefully grabbing his extremities. We tied them up to the stretcher rails so that he couldn't flail around and assault anyone else. It wasn't easy either, remember that super strength I told you about that comes to the mentally ill? Yeah, well that kicked in when he got pissed. An antipsychotic drug called haloperidol even had to be given to the patient to subdue him. Everything was under control shortly after we gave him the haloperidol. Our patient stayed nice and calm until the ER doors automatically slid open and he thought he had arrived at a show that he was the star of. He looked around at everyone with his arms outstretched wide and said, "Hellloooo Everybodieeesss!! The Burger King is here!!"

The way of the wicked is an abomination unto the Lord: but he loveth him that followeth after righteousness. **Proverbs 15:9**

#14

High Sugar Level Turned Sweet Tooth

Paramedic Pointer» *The culprit to an unconscious person may be low blood sugar. If you know the individual to be a diabetic, don't hesitate to check their blood sugar if you know how, it speeds up the diagnoses before EMS arrives. Normal ranges are between 70-120 mg/dL.*

Diabetic patients generally have two kinds of problems when they phone 911. One of two things is usually going on and they are: low blood sugar or high blood sugar. Both are dangerous because a low enough blood sugar level can make a person unconscious. The human brain essentially needs sugar to function properly, but keep in mind that sugar, though essential to brain functionality, is only one of many components needed. On the opposite end of the spectrum is the issue of having a ridiculously high blood sugar level. A dangerous condition called ketoacidosis can arise when an individual's blood sugar breaches a certain level. Diabetic ketoacidosis causes unsavory symptoms such as weakness or fatigue, nausea/vomiting, shortness of breath and confusion.

Though *this* particular patient's blood sugar was very high, it was not high enough for diabetic ketoacidosis to set in. However, this particular patient did throw Jeff and I for a loop by having what I refer to as developing a sweet tooth. She was a 21-year-old female patient who was found at a doctor's clinic. Her name was Caroline, she was Caucasian. When Jeff and I walked into the walk-in clinic to meet Caroline initially, she was quiet and shy, slow to respond and didn't say much. Accompanied by her mother, it was explained to us that she had experienced diabetic complications before. Today, her issue was fatigue, nausea and abdominal pain. Inside the clinic we manually obtained Caroline's vital signs to get a baseline before moving her out to the truck. Using our glucometer (a device used to record a blood sugar level) we obtained an initial sugar reading. Caroline's blood sugar was exceptionally high, a potential risk that needed to be further evaluated at the hospital, especially with Caroline having multiple symptoms. The ambulance doors shut, leaving only myself, Caroline and Jeff in each other's company at this point. Jeff took a seat in the captain's chair (the chair that sits directly behind the patient's head — usually for the paramedic writing the report) and I prepared my IV set up on the bench seat. Jeff began to ask pertinent questions to Caroline as I obtained another set of vital signs before applying a tourniquet. It is standard to apply a tourniquet when doing IVs because it helps the patients veins to "show themselves" better. Caroline's eyes began to wander around the ambulance as if she was pondering something. She took the IV like a champ, not budging or complaining one bit through the process.

Caroline bit her bottom lip and smirked in a mischievous manner upon me completing the IV in her left forearm. "Which one of you will be riding back here with me when we get to the hospital?" Caroline asked with a now devilish grin. Jeff and I immediately gave one another a raised eyebrow. We both had deemed that question to be quite interesting — we had never been asked that one before. "Uhh, I will be sitting back here to monitor you," Jeff said. We often alternated driving and tending to the patient in the back — it happened to be my turn to drive this call. Caroline quickly asked my name. I answered. Caroline's shoulders dropped in disappointment and she said, "Ahhh Fooey! Me want Lorenzo to sit in the back with me! Me love Lorenzo!" Weirdly enough, she didn't say it in an adult voice, but rather in a baby voice. It was almost as if she had two personalities because the voice she spoke in now was completely animated. "Me love Lorenzo! Me love Lorenzo! Me love Lorenzo!" She chanted in an impatient blitz. Jeff had even tried to say something but she cut him off, chanting, "me don't want Jeff! Me want Lorenzo! Me love Lorenzo!"

"I love Lorenzo too, Jeff said, but Lorenzo has got to drive on this call. You'll see him at the hospital and you can have allllll the Lorenzo you want. I'll even leave you two alone when we get there so you can have some time to yourselves," he finished, with an evil smile while looking at me. Diluting Caroline's high blood sugar with fluids through the IV was a temporary solution, which we did employ. But like many patients, Caroline needed blood labs done to measure her different enzymes in order to find imbalances and would likely need an insulin treatment. In leaving Caroline at the hospital, she remained her flirtatious, baby-talking self. I wished her well as the Doc came in to replace me at her bedside.

*The Lord thy God in the midst of thee is mighty; he will save, he will rejoice over thee with joy; he will rest in his love, he will joy over thee with singing. **Zephaniah 3:17***

#15

I'll Huff And I'll Puff

Paramedic Pointer» *People get high as a means of escapism many times because they are unhappy with their personal lives. Take note that whether you go to sleep or get high as an act of rebellion, you are still the same person when you return from your escape.*

I gotta tell you, there is all sorts of people who are into all kinds of mischief. Sometimes the mischief even happens in broad daylight — right in front of the public. On a busy street, a spot with high traffic isn't where you'd expect someone to be intoxicating themselves — not someone who doesn't want to get caught anyway. There are a large percentage of people, however, who are so lost in their addiction or vice that they tend to set all rational thinking to the side. This statement was irrefutably true for a blond haired woman who sat under a large oak tree. Next to her were four bottles of duster leaned up against a fence, just as she was. The blond haired woman looked like crap; it really was a pitiful situation to behold. Her hair had all sorts of leaves and debris in it. She had what paramedics refer to as "raccoon eyes" which is two black eyes that signify significant head trauma. Her mouth contained "summer teeth" — summer there and summer not. This poor female was trashed. You don't find an attractive woman in this predicament much — at least not on the side of the road.

Though beat up and bruised, one could still see her beauty shine through the ugliness that had stricken her. Jeff and I approached the completely drained woman who was resting up against the fence beneath the tree. Our district chief happened to respond to this particular call and was already on scene having an investigative conversation with her. "Hey guys," our district chief turned and greeted Jeff and I. "This is Michelle," she has been out here for about an hour now. She refuses to let go of the duster, which she has been huffing on for the duration of her picnic under this tree," he facetiously informed us. "Aaannd... That's how far I got until you all showed up," he added. I acknowledged his brief history given on the patient while turning towards her, "It's time to get up and come with us to the hospital miss Michelle," I exclaimed. She shook her head up and down in agreement before slowly rising to her feet. I was happy to see that Michelle was not resisting because due to her being under the influence, so to speak, she did not qualify to sign a refusal — that is a luxury offered to stable patients who are mentally competent. We typically gauge mental alertness with a term called A&O times 4. This stands for alert and oriented times four. It refers to an individual being aware of four things: person, place, time and event.

Michelle fooled me into thinking she was going to cooperate with her initial submissive behavior. It did not take long for her impulsive behavior to come out. Everything was going smoothly in buckling her into the stretcher with our safety belts (just like a car seat belt). Something possessed Michelle in an instant because she ripped off the belts, jumped off of the stretcher and sprinted back to her cans of duster. In doing so, she nearly fell, stumbling over one of the oak tree's above ground roots. Snatching one can of duster, Michelle threw her head back and huffed away; her eyes rolled into the back of her head, she conveyed an image of demonic satisfaction as if she was receiving supernatural power from the can of duster. Jeff, the district chief and I all grabbed her to escort her back to the cot. She went along with it for a moment, only to tear away from the grips of Jeff and the district chief's. Now she had one hand free. Michelle gave it all she had in leaping towards the cans with an outstretched arm to get one last huff. I pulled back on her arm — the one I had control of, but Michelle dove out just far enough to reach her beloved can. Just as she prepared to take another hit of the duster, the district chief knocked the can out of her hand with a downward slap of brute force. "We can't have you doing that Michelle!" The district chief raised his voice in authority. "Now come on already so we can check you out!" He continued.

Finally, we successfully loaded Michelle into the ambulance. The DC (District Chief) took off once we got her into the truck— another call came in that he left to respond to. The basics, as far as Michelle's breathing rate, heart rate and blood pressure were doing well, they were all within normal limits. Our patient's light twitching was of concern, however— "Why are you shaking like that?" I asked. "I need a cigarette, it will calm my nerves," she replied. "I hear you, but that can't happen while you're being medically evaluated," I told her. Michelle just stared at the rear ambulance wall with a slight grin— I can't tell you *why* she was grinning. "Do you have any children?" I inquired. "Yes, I have four little ones and I had a husband…" She said with an odd look on her face. "Well what happened to your husband, Michelle?" I asked with compassion. "He died two weeks ago from an overdose," she said casually. It was almost as if it was not a devastating event in her life. She spoke of it as if it was only some sort of mild occurrence that happened to have unraveled. "Where are your children?" I asked. "Oh, they're being watched by my brother right now. He will have them for a couple of hours." "All so you can come out here and do this, right??" Jeff impatiently joked. "… Yes," Michelle reluctantly answered with her head down. "My oldest of the four is 10 years old. He's pretty much aware that his mommy has a problem, but he's the only one of my children who is on to me," she said with guilt. "With one of your kids already aware of what you're doing, don't you think it'd be a smart idea to really try and stop?" Jeff questioned her. "Yes… I do… I'm going to stop," Michelle responded. She said it in a way that made one believe she sincerely planned to stop. It's just too bad that this particular day would not be the day Michelle quit. Jeff and I transported her to the hospital safely. Later that shift, we were informed by our DC that Michelle had been transported to the hospital four times that day for the same exact thing.

And all thy children shall be taught of the Lord; and great shall be the peace of thy children. **Isaiah 54:13**

#16

Terrible Twos

Paramedic Pointer» *Place all prescription pills high enough and out of sight of toddlers because they are fearless explorers at this age, looking for opportunity to experiment. Remove cleaning chemicals from their reach as well. The colorful liquid may appear as a "tasty drink" in a toddler's eyes.*

They often refer to year two in a toddler's life as the "terrible twos" because this is the age toddler's run around putting things in their mouth and tear things up. They view themselves as great explorers — and they are. Everything is so new to a two-year-old. They have got to touch, taste and even swallow anything they can get their little paws on. Accidents happen. Inevitably, accidents are going to occur, as more seasoned individuals (parents and guardians), we should work hard at minimizing neglecting certain responsibilities — starting with placing prescription meds in a high, secured place so that the little ones running around the house don't mistake it for candy. One mother left an open container of pills open that almost resulted in her toddler's death.

Around 10 AM, we were headed to a call in a more rural area concerning the well-being of a two-year-old. Entering the front door segued a terrified mother screaming at the top of her lungs. It was a young blonde mother with a bob haircut. She was still in her pajamas, having only a tank top on and short shorts on that had a pink flower on them. Her son— the two-year-old— sat on the bed appearing severely fatigued. Drowsy is probably the precise word to describe his condition because the toddler sat upright with his head intermittently dropping down and around in circles. If you've ever seen someone fighting to stay awake in a chair that keeps falling asleep, then you could imagine the state this toddler was in. "Is he going to be okay?! Is my baby going to be okay?!" The young mother cried out hysterically. I rushed over to the little guy and felt the quality of his pulse — strong. The temperature felt normal upon touching his forehead and neck which were positive signs. He was warm, not hot or cold.

Other vital signs proved to be decent so the next thing I thought about was why the toddler couldn't seem to stay awake. By this time, a cop had walked over and notified me that mommy left her prescribed *Subutex* open on the floor by mistake, according to her. Subutex is medication given to people addicted to narcotics in order to help wean them off. "Oh no," I thought instantly. Mommy being an addict with a small child was scary enough, but the fact that her son had actually ingested Subutex pills left an eerie feeling in the pit of my stomach that lingered. Fear of the unknown caused multiple thoughts to race through my head.

For starters, pediatric patients always receive medication in weight-based doses, but Subutex was not on the list of meds toddler's take. After all, what two-year-old have you ever known to be addicted to narcotics? Kids are certainly maturing quite fast these days, it seems, but for Pete's sake, not that fast. When we transport a pediatric patient, we have to use an approved car seat that we are given by our agency. Jeff set the car seat up on our cot, strapping it into the cot so it did not move around. As soon as we placed the toddler on the pediatric seat he began to vomit clear fluid. It trickled down his chin and onto his little pop belly. As you may imagine, the mother, who had managed to calm herself down moments ago, was now hysterical again. "What's going on?! What's wrong with him?! Look at him! He's throwing up!!" Mommy yelled as she covered her mouth with one hand and pointed with her other. She looked pale as if she was sentenced to death. "Your son vomiting isn't a bad thing sweetheart," Jeff explained to mommy. "It's a good thing that he's clearing all of that medicine out of his system," Jeff explained further. In hearing this, mommy simmered back down, collecting her supercharged nerves once again. The toddler's mother sat on the bench seat in the back of the ambulance to accompany her child.

Whenever possible, this was done to prevent small children from freaking out. We never want a small child to feel as though he or she is being kidnapped — which is the reaction when a parent is not present. Ambulance rides are fearful experiences for many adults, let alone for a toddler. Climbing into a gigantic truck with all sorts of gadgets and gizmos is downright intimidating for many toddlers.

The transport went smooth; I wish I could say the same for the actual handoff at the hospital. For some reason, a nursed stepped away from the ER room the toddler was being monitored in. The nurse did state that the mother of the two-year-old patient was in the room watching her son — and had agreed to not go anywhere while the nurse was running a quick errand. I was changing the sheets on our stretcher when a desperate voice came from the toddler's hospital room… "I'm gonna need a nurse…NOW!!" An ER medic panicked. Half of the ER must have rushed into the room, including myself. Our two-year-old patient suddenly lost consciousness, turning purple in the face. Assisted ventilations were started seconds after the ER medic called for help — shortly after the assisted ventilations were initiated, the two-year-old regained both his color and his consciousness. He began to cry, segueing a simultaneous sigh of relief from everyone in the room. Crying from a baby means that he or she has a patent or "open" airway which is of optimal concern. Now the narcotic addicted mother had returned from a smoke break, bathroom break or wherever she went and returned with a red hot temper. "What's wrong with you people?!" She snapped at the nurse who told her she was stepping away for a moment. The nurse gave mommy clear instructions to not leave until she returned. Go figure. Needless to say, mommy was escorted out of the room by security. The nurse broke down in tears because she was stricken with the false guilt that it was all her fault. I consoled her briefly until my radio on my hip let off a loud tone followed by "medic 16 respond to…" It was time to skedaddle — that was us.

*But whoso looketh into the perfect law of liberty, and continueth therein, he being not a forgetful hearer, but a doer of the work, this man shall be blessed in his deed. **James 1:25***

#17

Hyperventilater On Weedon Island

Paramedic Pointer» *When you hyperventilate fast enough (usually during a panic attack) you can exhale so much carbon dioxide that your hands lock up into bawled fists. Try to remain calm at all times and regulate your breathing.*

Weedon Island was a beautiful island where people would ride their bikes on the available trail, take in the sights or use the Gulf to do recreational water activities. It was offset from the mainlands, providing for a good escape from the inner city congestion and chaos. Florida sunshine illuminated the entire island quite nicely on this day, giving every rock and tree a brilliant golden glow to it. People who were jogging or biking were affected by the rays too, receiving golden tater tot tans. Due to the geographical location of Weedon Island, our ambulance response time was longer than usual. We first had to make it to the island; secondly, we had to make it *through* the big Island. Filled with numerous twists and turns, short winding roads had our vast ambulance doing a serpentine dance. Our patient's location turned out to be in the very back of the island, typical for our luck. No joke, every time Jeff and I got a call at a nursing home; it was the last room at the end of the hallway. We'd like to be able to say our luck changed with the change of environment, but it didn't. Not even a little bit. It was inevitably the furthest point in any vicinity we responded to — every single time. A waver on the edge of the road where sand met concrete stood there in excitement. A waver is a person literally outside waving the ambulance down so that we don't bypass our target.

Anyways, this aided us in stopping at just the right spot along the sandy shore. There were a multitude of trees in the area, providing a great deal of shade. Water gently splashed up against a soggy shoreline. Slowly drawing toward the shore was a freaked out male breathing rapidly and a worried look-ing female sitting behind him rowing the kayak. She was the only one of the two rowing because the man was frozen in place— he was as stiff as a dead person. Their kayak gently came to a halt on the mushy sand just before Jeff and I stepped in for a closer look. The woman wasted no time in explaining what happened. "We were out kayaking in the Gulf for about 30 minutes when my fiancé started to get tired. He began breathing faster and faster until he began hyperventilating. I tried to calm him down, you know, coach him out of a panic attack and his hands locked up. It's so strange! I knew he wasn't in the best of shape, but I didn't think this would happen," the patient's fiancé explained. "I work out a lot more than him so I'm in much better shape than him," she boasted casually. We all had an uneasy laugh about that comment.

Switching the focus back to the man, he was still helplessly frozen. A look of sheer terror was plastered on his face. His fists were clenched tighter than someone curling heavy dumbbells. "What's his name?" we asked his fiancé. He was in such shock that Jeff, nor I, bothered to even direct the question at him, who appeared indefinitely mute. "His name is Brian," the fiancé replied in a hurried fashion. "Brian, I'm gonna need you to try your hardest to focus with me. Slow your breathing down because your rapid breaths are causing you to blow off too much carbon dioxide. This is what's causing you to lock up the way that you are," I said in a loud, directive tone. Brian slowly forced his head to turn towards me, still frozen with a horrific look on his face as if someone had scared the crap out of him. He was pale as well — his skin took on a faded complexion that only contributed to the overall appearance of the shock he displayed. "Breathe nice and slow, deep breaths. Nice and slow, nice and slow," I coached Brian. Little by little, he managed to decrease his breathing rate.

Brian's eyes instantly switched from focusing on me to his hands, which he realized were coming back under his control. They slowly uncurled from the death clench he had just moments ago.

Jeff applied a nasal cannula to help deliver supplemental oxygen to aid Brian's breathing. If you've ever seen those light green or clear colored tubes that fit snug inside hospital patients' nose, then you know what a nasal cannula is. Brian gave an expression of relief, his shoulders dropping down what seemed to be about 6 inches. In applying a capnography cannula (a cannula that measures exhaled carbon dioxide), Brian's numbers were now within normal limits. I started an IV to give Brian some fluids because he was a bit dehydrated. His pale, discoloration returned to him during transport to the ER. No other problems were present so it was smooth sailing from here on out with Brian, a lot smoother than his kayak scare.

Not everyone that saith unto me, Lord, Lord, shall enter into the kingdom of heaven; but he that doeth the will of my father which is in heaven. **Matthew 7:21**

#18

What Are The Odds?

Paramedic Pointer» *In cases of allergic reactions, an over the counter drug that can be administered is 25-50mg of Benadryl. It is an antihistamine which combats allergic reactions. Further, Benadryl has sedative properties in it, which is why you may find yourself dosing off shortly after ingestion.*

Ever find yourself asking, "What are the odds of this happening?" On a perfectly normal day out on Anna Maria Island, I found myself asking the same question. A young girl, about 14 years old, was reported to have breathing problems with an "abnormal appearance". Beach crowds on the weekends in Florida tend to be packed, but we had no trouble spotting this young girl because she stuck out like a sore thumb. She stood by the beach restrooms, resembling a bright red, cartoon blowfish. Tears were cascading down her meaty cheeks and she was bouncing up and down slightly, shaking her hands, as if she had to use the bathroom. What must've been her mother ran up to Jeff and I when we got off the truck in a rush to give us the rundown. "She can't breathe! Her throat is swollen! She almost passed out! I think she stepped on a bee, there was a stinger in her foot that we took out!" The anonymous woman cried out in one big breath. This was the part where I asked that question to myself that I mentioned earlier. This was that moment I experienced what I'm sure we've all had at one time in our lives. The patient was barefoot, as expected, for someone spending time at the beach. Her being barefoot certainly contributed to her vulnerability to this *longshot*.

Nonetheless, it happened. We were there and we were ready to help. Our patient was clearly experiencing *angioedema*, a condition where pretty much your entire face gets swollen — including your airway. Her face looked inflated like a balloon. Eyelids swollen, lips and throat swollen upon evaluating the inside of her mouth, her tongue took up every bit of space in her throat there was — leaving none at all. All she could do was try to breathe out of her nostrils. Jeff drew up the dosages of epinephrine and Benadryl. I quickly looked for a usable vein to start a line in (IV). Wrapping the tourniquet tightly around her upper arm, decent veins began to expose themselves. I needed to clean the IV site with an alcohol prep pad. Up popped a perfect vein— in a very short time— to my satisfaction. I successfully threaded the needle catheter into her impressive blood vessel. "Here you are," Jeff said to me, extending his drawn up dosage of Benadryl. Jeff administered the epinephrine in the patient's deltoid (shoulder muscle).

Moving quickly, our patient's blood pressure and pulse was taken. Her pulse was elevated; her blood pressure was low. She was in anaphylactic shock — a crisis where one's blood pressure gets abnormally low from having a severe allergic reaction. She would need fluids soon to get her blood pressure back up to par. About two minutes after medication administration, the young girl's symptoms subsided. It was as if someone poked a hole in a balloon and all the air had escaped. Her face generally maintained a full appearance but swelling in her lips, throat, eyes and tongue went down tremendously—throat and tongue being most important due to airway clearance. Our patient progressed from a panic to a relaxed state in little time. Her flushed red appearance went away as well. "Now that we've got all that swelling down and you can breathe, may I ask your name miss?" I began to establish rapport. "Megan", the young girl replied. "Something told me I shouldn't have walked through that grassy area with no sandals on", she said with a frown. "Yeah no kidding, it's too bad you didn't follow your gut instinct on that one. Isn't it ironic how fast things can turn from normal to chaotic in a split second?" I joked. "The good news is that everything is now under control. You should be glad because you're lucky enough to get the all-stars today, Jeff and I are the county's finest", I boasted with a smile. The young patient enjoyed my light humor, but quickly withdrew back into a nervous demeanor.

Not being able to breathe is no joking matter, the fear that her airway swelling would rekindle was probably discomforting her. Airway difficulties give off a sense of impending doom — after all, you are flirting with suffocation. Years ago, I personally experienced anaphylaxis (severe allergic reaction with difficulty breathing). Being an irresponsible, non-attentive teenager, led to me not taking my anti-histamine before going in for an allergy treatment. An anti-histamine (Benadryl for example) stops a person from having a bad reaction to the allergy treatment. Essentially what the treatment entails is injecting the person being treated with small doses of what they are *already* allergic to. Without the antihistamine, big trouble can occur. I was on the way home that day when I strangely began coughing up huge mucus plugs, repeatedly spitting them out of the driver side window on the way home. Eventually my throat closed up about 90%. When I got to my house I thrashed the countertops in my kitchen as well as the tops of all my bedroom dressers. I was desperately in search of my much needed antihistamine. Epinephrine would have been appropriate too but I didn't have any. I'm here so you know I found my medication that day. But anyhow, Megan took an easy ride with us down to the hospital to be further evaluated. She extended a hearty thank you to Jeff and I for intervening on her crisis so speedily. "All we wanted was to keep you breathing, you're too young to check out already," Jeff joked, referring to death in a roundabout way.

For ye have need of patience, that, after ye have done the will of God, ye might receive the promise. **Hebrews 10:36**

#19

Brenda The Building Jumper

Paramedic Pointer» *Risperdal, Valproic acid, Zoloft, Seroquel— to name a few— are psychiatric medications. This will give you clues of what type of company you are in if these medications are spotted in a person's possession.*

B renda wound up being the highlight of my Thanksgiving one year instead of a turkey. I decided to pull a 12-hour overtime shift because my agency, at the time, paid double time and a half on Thanksgiving. My ambulance was riding three deep because our third person was a newbie being trained. It was myself, a paramedic named Jeremy and the new girl, whose name I cannot recall — she will be referred to as "new girl" in this story. This shift was completely an off-the-cuff decision to work; The night before I saw an opening for the 0400 – 1600 shift. I figured it was a win-win move to make with being able to still make it home to family in time for a turkey dinner. As I mentioned already, double time and a half was being paid out too, so that also influenced my decision. Normally I'm with my partner Jeff, but today I was a part of a trio. Jeremy was an extremely smart paramedic. He was also extremely flamboyant. He was an average size man with gray hair and wore reading glasses. He could tell you about a slew of minor details most paramedics did not pay much attention to in regards to prehospital management. Jeremy was a veteran with our agency.

New girl was very well kept. She was neat, having creases in her uniform sleeves, creases in her uniform pants and a golden watch to match her golden hair she wore in a bun. Her nails were done in the French tip style. The overall vibe she gave off was "prissy", which was atypical to the common rugged female paramedic. Little did we know we were all going to experience a special patient to help us remember this Thanksgiving by.

Our patient was being kept at a psychiatric facility called PEMHS (pronounced "pems"). Sitting in their small lobby, our patient waited for direction with her legs crossed. A facility representative came out and debriefed us. "She's very excitable, she has not been known to get physical, but she does say outrageous things," the woman transferring care told us. I don't mean to sound too harsh, but our patient looked atrocious. Her name was Brenda, and boy was Brenda one disgusting lump of DNA. Smelling of dumpster contents, she looked also as if she crawled out of a sewer. Her teeth were completely rotted. Her hair had enough debris in it for a large bird to mistake it for a nest. Her nails looked as if they had never been cleaned in her life. So she sat there in silence while her paperwork was being prepared. It didn't take long before we were asking Brenda to stand and pivot on to our cot. Brenda did just as we asked, all the while with a devious grin on her face. She looked as if she had something in store for us — a hidden agenda that was currently being kept secret. I knew she had a mischievous plan; it would not take long before her evil plot was revealed. History shows that with psychiatric patients, it never does take long. Right when the three of us paramedics rolled Brenda out of PEMHS is when the fun began (I say that facetiously). Brenda sized each of us up while slowly rubbing her hands together. "WHAT ARE YOU LOOKING AT YOU LITTLE WHORE?! YOU THINK YOU'VE GOT EVERYONE FOOLED, DON'T YOU, YOU LITTLE SLUT!?!?" Brenda said to new girl. New girl did not let it phase her composure, maintaining her posture. "THAT'S WHAT I THOUGHT YOU MUTT!" Brenda said, salivating from her mouth.

Next, she tried her hand at Jeremy, who was directly behind her head with two hands on the stretcher, pushing it along. Brenda burst out with a now demon possessed voice. First, she shot an evil eye at me and barked,

"JUST LOOK AT YOU! YOU'RE NOTHING BUT A PATHETIC PIMP! AND THIS FLAMING FAGOT BEHIND ME IS A TINKERBELL, I OUGHTTA SHOVE THIS STRETCHER UP HIS A**!!!" Brenda seemed to have a bipolar/Tourette's duo going on psychologically. Jeremy shook his head slowly behind the head of the stretcher as he continued to push it forward. "Hey, happy Thanksgiving to you too Miss Brenda", Jeremy replied in a joking fashion. Lifting Brenda (while on the stretcher) into the back of the ambulance, the three of us paramedics gave each other a look that said, "Here we go" without words. When I placed the blood pressure cuff on our patient she turned on her seductive voice and asked me, "You're a good boy aren't you?" While slowly nodding her head up and down as if to help me in giving her the right answer. She smiled at me with those rotted teeth which were barely discernible to even be teeth at this point in her life. Brenda had on a super faded black T-shirt and black basketball shorts. She began feeling herself up with a twisted smirk on her face while doing so. "Oh would you just stop Brenda? That is disgusting!" Jeremy snapped. Brenda's sexually inappropriate behavior went on for the duration of the transport to our destination. She was to be seen at Indian rocks Hospital, a hospital with a dedicated sector for psychiatric patients. Though she remained in her sexual mode, collecting our needed vital signs was a breeze for the most part. We unloaded the stretcher (with Brenda on it of course).

The sexually inappropriate behavior peaked on our way to the elevator. In the long hallway, she found it necessary to pull out one of her large, floppy breasts and wave it around carelessly. "What are you doing Brenda? That is just gross, now stop it!" Jeremy scolded her. Brenda stopped and became calm all of a sudden. Entering the elevator, she again asked me if I was a good boy. "Why don't you take me up to the top of this building and jump off the top with me while holding hands? Wouldn't that be so romantic?" She asked me with her head tilted sideways. Glancing at the elevator buttons, there were 17 floors. I remained neutral to her psychopathic advances. Doing so gave Brenda nothing to feed off of. She changed direction once she found that she had nothing to run with from me. She was seeking a "rise" out of someone. If she could just get one of us riled up she would be entertained. Realizing that she was most successful in doing so with Jeremy, she continued to brutally antagonize Jeremy anyway she could. "YOU'RE MOTHER WAS A CRACK WHORE WHO NEVER LOVED YOU!" Brenda violently insulted. Turning the first corner following our exit from the elevator brought into view a huge sign mounted above the door that read "psychiatric unit". There was a security clearance panel to the right of the entrance door where a badge needed to be scanned. A doctor opened the door for us once he saw us through the small square window.

Brenda was thrashing around on the stretcher. The Doc, who had on the common long white coat gave her an aggravated stare, one that conveyed a no tolerance demeanor. It was a look that expressed how often the Doc dealt with this behavior. "Draw up the Geodon," he told a psychiatric nurse. The Doc's eyes stayed glued on Brenda until the nurse returned with the syringe filled with Geodon. Geodon is an antipsychotic medication given to treat mental conditions such as bipolar, schizophrenia and Tourette's syndrome. The nurse handed over the syringe, which had a needle attached to it. The Doc finally took his eyes off of Brenda—but only for a split second. He pushed a few drops of medication out of the tip of the needle to ensure all of the air was out — pushing air into a patient can cause great complications up to and including death.

"WHERE IS MY ONE, TRUE LOVE?! IS HE COMING, IS HE COMING?!" Brenda said in her demonic voice. The Doc casually, yet purpose-fully, walked closer to Brenda. "No dear, Geodon is coming. "GEODON?" Brenda asked. "Yes… Geodon is coming dear," said the Doc. STICK!! The psychiatric doctor stuck the needle in her upper arm and injected the medica-tion. A minute or two later, Brenda slowly became weaker with drowsy eyes. No longer was she thrashing around on the cot, but rather laid there with no energy to expend. We unhooked Brenda from our wires and with help from a few psychiatric attendants, moved her over to the facility bed. Her eyes were the only thing left that had any fight left, but they were going in circles as if she was seeing stars. Brenda fought it until she could fight no more— until ever so gently, her eyes closed. Brenda had faded to black.

And the peace of God, which passeth all understanding, shall keep your hearts and minds through Christ Jesus. **Philippians 4:7**

#20

Underwater Sleeper

Paramedic Pointer» *People with Narcolepsy have trouble regulating sleep/wakefulness cycles— this is a brain dysfunction. The average person has the ability to wake up at a designated time, even without their alarm. This internal clock is called your circadian rhythm.*

The beautiful thing about Florida is that it's a peninsula, one side less attached to land and we'd be an island. In fact, Florida is the closest thing to an island in the states — and people love islands. People take cruises to the Bahamas every year for vacation. They plan weddings in the Cayman Islands all the time. Or how about the "just because" trips to exotic islands to go snorkeling or sightseeing. Being from St. Petersburg, Florida, I've been fortunate to have grown up in a place where you can touch water (ocean) if you simply travel 15 minutes in any direction. When I was attending Eckerd College my freshman year of college, I can remember my three good buddies, who were from New Jersey, Kentucky and Atlanta, feeling like they were in paradise. But as any commodity or perk in this world, having water around can sometimes turn negative. There's the boating accidents, shark bites, stingrays, dangerous waves, flood risks for beachfront properties, etc. And of course a term we've all been acclimated to hear every so often since the beginning of time — drownings — whether in a tub, a jacuzzi, a pool, or in the sea.

Jeff and I took a ride out to the beach — but not for our leisure. We'd sometimes eat breakfast at a beach restaurant but not today, this was no situation of laid back nature — someone had *drowned*. The way beach condominiums and resorts were set up on the beach coast was like a wall— every building so close together that it made seeing the ocean difficult in this particular area. Jeff and I were trying to spot where the scene was, but with no luck. Dispatch shot us a message on our mobile computer — the name of the resort our patient was behind. We pulled into the *Tradewinds* Beach resort and unpacked our stretcher out of the back of the ambulance. Our stretcher wheels are not large enough, nor are they made to roll efficiently in the sand, so this meant carrying our three heavy bags at least 100 yards in the sand until we reached the water. The blazing sun created an oven effect — it felt literally as if I was being baked. Our walk turned into a miniature hike. Every step we took sank deeply into the sand. Our heavy bags— about 40 pounds a piece— made us sink down even more. In our path appeared a downed man lying on his back, just beyond a mound of sand — we were almost there.

"We may have to take a dip in the ocean after this call," Jeff said referring to the scorching heat. I glanced over at Jeff to see his face drenched in sweat. I could even see big beads of sweat accumulating on his upper lip. Reaching the downed patient a few steps later, we quickly knelt down to lay hands on the older gentleman, who looked to be in his late 60s. "Can you feel a pulse?" Jeff asked me as I felt the patient's carotid artery on his neck. "Nothing," I immediately shot back. Marine rescue — the two-man crew who posted on the beach were lifeguards/paramedics, they were the ones who had pulled this older gentleman out of the ocean. "Let's begin CPR as soon as we place this backboard underneath him", I announced. Putting a rigid backboard underneath the patient during CPR made chest compressions more effective. One of the Marine medics began CPR after he slapped on the defibrillation pads. "I'll get an IV going and get some drugs on board (inside the patient) if you want to take care of the airway", I told Jeff as I broke out the life-saving medication box. There we were — just beyond the splash of the water riding up on the sandy shore, pumping away on the patient who was said to have been walking out into the water and fell forward. Beach calls are among the messiest of emergencies when it comes to cardiac arrest. Sand is everywhere. It's on you, it's on the patient, it's on your equipment (the worst) and it soon gets into your ambulance by default.

SHOCK!! First defibrillation delivered. That is, our patient had just received a jolt of electricity through his body. "STILL NO PULSE!!" I announced. Rotating chest compressors, the first marine medic backed away from the patient, allowing the second Marine medic to now do chest compressions. Another round of drugs was administered. "Come on man," I silently rooted for our patient in my head. SHOCK!! A second jolt of electricity surged through the patient's body. Jeff yelled, "DO WE HAVE A PULSE?!" checking...checking... "YES, WE HAVE A PULSE BACK!!" I answered as soon as I felt the faint thumping on my index and middle finger. "VERY NICE", Jeff acknowledged, starting to get up from his knees. We had attracted a huge crowd who slowly inched closer to us throughout the call to get a closer look. "EVERYONE SCOOT ON BACK SO THAT WE CAN MOVE AS QUICK AS POSSIBLE", Jeff instructed the audience. There was a marine unit that they were blocking. It was one of the vehicles with huge tires on it for driving in the sand, more or less sporty golf carts with monster wheels. It had space on the back to place a patient on, just like a pickup truck has a bed, so to speak, on the rear. Jeff hopped into the bed to keep the patient from sliding around in the vehicle and one of the two marine medics drove. The second marine medic and myself lugged the remaining equipment that could not fit into the beach vehicle.

We hauled butt as fast as we could to get back to the ambulance to link back up with the other two medics. We had to dig deep and hustle through the thick sand in order to not slow the process of transport. With our now revived patient, things were looking much brighter. He was still unconscious — not to mention with a tube down his throat receiving assisted ventilations — but he was *alive*.

Delivery was successfully made to the receiving hospital. It was later found that our guy had a history of narcolepsy and Parkinson's disease. His witnessed act of "falling forward" in the ocean water was likely him merely falling asleep. Approximately three days later, Jeff and I saw our narcoleptic patient in the

ER, fully alert. He was laying down in the hospital bed next to his wife, who sat in a chair holding his hand. "Hello sir", I said with a big smile on my face. Jeff did the same, standing next to me with a similar demeanor. "Hello there", the man replied, looking jovial. "Do you remember us?" Jeff asked. "Uhh… No… I don't believe I've ever seen you before", the man replied. "Do you remember anything at all? Or rather, what *is* the last thing you remember?" Jeff questioned, fishing to see how well his memory was — or if it was even present in regard to his near-death experience. "Let's see, the only thing I remember is walking out into the water… After that there was just black," the patient said. "So you don't even remember seeing myself or Jeff at any point that day?" I asked. "No… No I don't unfortunately… Who are you two fellas anyway?" He cheerfully questioned us. His wife interjected abruptly, saying, "John, these are the two young men who saved your life".

*He will be very gracious unto thee at the voice of thy cry; when he
shall hear it, he will answer thee.* **Isaiah 30:19**

#21

Pain, Pain Go Away!

Paramedic Pointer» *Being "allergic" to every pain medication
in the book except for the strongest narcotics isn't typical at all.
This is a red flag for caregivers, in fact. It strongly suggests a drug-
seeking patient.*

If you've ever met a junkie then you might be aware of how far they will go to
get a "fix". Virtues such as honesty, patience, loyalty, etc. tend to get put on
the back burner. Pride tends to take a backseat. And dignity, well, I'm not sure
if there's much of that left anywhere in the world these days. First and fore-
most, there is a great benefit to pain medication — narcotics to be exact. They
reduce discomfort and increase our threshold for pain tolerance — what's not
to like? The problem lies in the seldom recipient that gets some for a legitimate
cause and wants more. Not just a little more, not just more until the pain
goes away either. I'm talking more as in the desire for a *lifetime's* worth of pain
meds. They spend much of their precious time plotting, scheming, conjuring,
distorting, faking, frolicking, fretting and fearing that they won't get their precious narcotics again. As with anything there is a good and a bad. A positive
and a negative. There is dark and also there is light. There's something to be
said about that old Ying and Yang concept isn't there? It's everywhere.

On this particular call I had been a probationary fire medic, working
alongside a fairly new fire medic named Trevor. We had the privilege to meet a

woman named Rochelle, who was lying in bed that day and what she *claimed* to be excruciating pain. She laid there with covers upon covers toppled over her body. Only her head was visible. Rochelle made it clear to us that she had fibromyalgia and lupus. She even educated us on every last symptom regarding pain they both entail. Something told me she was building an imaginary case to score some hardcore drugs. I casually approached her and asked if I could feel her pulse. She slowly took her left arm out from under the covers and extended it above the comforter. She rested her arm there with her palm facing the ceiling. I touched her wrist to assess her pulse and she began screaming at the top of her lungs about how bad it hurt to even be touched. "What's going on Rochelle?" I asked in a hurry. I had never had such a response when touching a patient with my mere fingertips! "I'm in pain! Touching me is unbearably painful!" She yelled. Rochelle began shaking her head side to side vigorously, appearing as to tell someone "no" without words. "Rochelle, I'm gonna need to touch you so that I can assess a few things hun," I calmly explained to her. She gritted her teeth and nodded in approval. Lightly touching her wrist for a second time, I noted that her pulse was strong and normal. Upon taking her blood pressure, it was within normal limits as well. "Where exactly do you hurt, Rochelle?" I asked. "EVERYWHERE! ALL OVER!!" The patient replied. I glanced over at Trevor to see if he was getting a weird vibe like I was. He seemed to be pondering what course of action to take from here. "MAKE THE PAIN STOP!" Rochelle prompted us. "What kind of medications do you take?" I responded. Rochelle informed us that she wasn't currently taking any. "Are you allergic to any meds?" I questioned further. Our patient instantly gave a look of slight nervousness, appearing as if this was the final question she needed to answer correctly in order to win the grand prize on a game show. "My allergies?" Rochelle asked, seeming to need some time to collect her thoughts. "... I'm allergic to codeine, oxycodone, Demerol, tramadol, morphine and Dilaudid," she said with absolute confidence. This list she recited sent up a red flag in my head — a big, vibrant red flag. See, Rochelle cleverly listed every pain medication that we didn't have on our truck except for one. We did have morphine, which she listed, but ironically the only drug she left out was *fentanyl*. Fentanyl, by the way, happens to be stronger than morphine anyway. Imagine that. Our lovely patient could only tolerate our strongest available drug. How convenient for her.

By this time, I was onto her schematic behavior, only, my other fellow paramedics on scene did not seem to catch on. I discreetly motioned Trevor to meet me just outside the bedroom in the hallway. "I believe we've got a faker on our hands. She seems to be trying to score drugs for personal pleasure", I whispered. "I was kind of thinking that but it's a hard one to call", Trevor whispered back in the hallway. "Hey, I'm on probation so that's your call, just wanted to bounce that idea off of you," I said. My experience had revealed a common thread among the drug-seeking community. They all seem to know which narcotics our ambulance kept on board. Therefore, they knew which pain meds to magically be allergic to because we paramedics don't administer drugs patients are allergic to. It leaves the drug they are after (in Rochelle's case it's Fentanyl) wide open for selection. An additional red flag is that Rochelle did not want her pain meds administered via IV, but intranasally (up her nose), which was unique to fentanyl. Fentanyl, unlike most other narcotic pain meds, can be given through the vein or up the nostrils. Average patients aren't aware of this fact, so Rochelle suggesting this made the red flag in my mind even brighter. Trevor drew up the fentanyl and gave it to me to shoot up her nose. When Rochelle saw this, she suddenly became like a dog before they get their treat. I could almost see a tail wagging behind her. I crawled into her king-sized bed and held the syringe to her right nostril and pushed the medication. Rochelle's eyes rolled into the back of her skull in satisfaction as she snorted every drop of the fentanyl. She took a few short snorts after the syringe was empty to make sure she didn't waste any. Rochelle was now satisfied, it was blatantly written all over her tanned face. She straightened out her face to appear neutral again because even she realized that she was giving herself away. You could tell it took a real effort to do, what she really wanted to do was bask in the glory of "cloud nine" but there were too many eyes on her.

Next came the ultimate giveaway— Trevor asked our female patient how she would like us to move her over to our stretcher. "I don't want to go to the hospital," she said, trying earnestly to nip the offer in the bud. "Well, uh, that's just not an option Rochelle," Trevor started explaining through a chuckle.

"See, once we give you a narcotic, it's against the law to leave a patient home. So in other words, you *will* be coming with us… So again, how would you like us to move you over to our stretcher? You can roll from the bed onto it, we can move you by lifting your body, or we can use a sheet," he explained. Trevor had now clearly seen the manipulation for what it was. Rochelle wanting to stay home after being given a powerful narcotic revealed her true plan. Rochelle was arrogant enough to think we were going to show up, give her a high and leave her unattended. Maybe it wasn't arrogance. Maybe it was her blissful ignorance to our standing protocols. The fact of the matter is that either way, she figured she could get away with it. And maybe she would have if it wasn't for narcotics being strong enough to kill someone, providing an unexpected occurrence such as an adverse reaction — which is basically a reaction that is far outside of the norm.

Rochelle tried to stall by talking our ears off, but had no success in changing the outcome. We chose the method of moving her to be by way of the sheet she was already laying on. Rochelle hollered the entire transfer from her bed to the stretcher. Neighbors probably were under the impression that she was being beaten to death or eaten alive by cannibals — that's how dramatic she was. And to top it off, Rochelle gave resisting transport one last go. On the way into the back of the ambulance, Rochelle spread her arms as wide as possible, grasping onto the side safety handles with a death grip. "NOOOO!!! YOU'RE NOT TAKING ME! YOU'RE NOT TAKING ME!!" Two firemen pried her fingers off of the safety handles, pushed the cot all the way inside the back of the truck and closed the doors behind her.

*The Lord is far from the wicked: but he heareth the prayer of the righteous. **Proverbs 15:29***

#22

Burned By The Boat

Paramedic Pointer» *Never smoke near an oxygen source, oxygen is flammable! One patient I treated decided to do this and it blew up in his face; he looked like the cartoon characters after they get blown up with dynamite.*

Boats don't typically burn people. A spilled cup of coffee, stove accident or traditional fire is commonplace. As for pediatrics, irons and other hot objects are concerns for toddlers running around the house. Safety pamphlets issued by health and public safety agencies will often remind you to be very responsible with these items for the sake of children — no one wants little four-year-old Jimmy knocking the hot iron onto him and getting seared. Some of the territory that comes with this job is witnessing common ways people tend to get injured, as well as the not so common ways.

Jeff and I responded to a boat marina in the middle of the summer. At this marina were some of the most impressive boats I had ever laid my eyes on. Being a Florida native, it wasn't my first time seeing a boat marina either— there are tons in the sunshine state. Next to this marina was a boating dock, where riders would get on and off their boat. Upon arriving on scene there were people getting off of a boat at the dock, leading Jeff and I to believe, briefly, that these were our patients. Something wasn't right. These particular people were all too elated— No sign of distress there. Our call notes disclosed that a 28-year-old female had been burned. Scanning the lot meticulously, no suspect was found. The area outside of the boat marina was more or less desolate… until a cry was heard. It was coming from inside the marina bay — where many boats were "garage kept", so to speak.

Rushing to the inside of the bay, we ran into six people, four guys and two girls. The four guys were carrying a young female, whose left leg was almost smoking from third-degree burns. "It hurts soooo bad! Somebody help meeee!" the female being carried cried. This clearly was our patient. The second girl was walking alongside the four guys carrying our patient with both hands covering her mouth — whose bottom jaw would have dropped all the way to the floor, by the way, had she not had her hands placed where they were. "You've got to do something…FAST! She was standing behind our boat when the engine exploded on her leg! Look at it!" One of the four guys exclaimed. They placed the burning patient on our stretcher and one (I assume was her boyfriend) gave her a goodbye kiss on the cheek. She was experiencing so much pain that I'm pretty sure she was totally numb and unaware of the gesture. "AHHHHHHH!" Her high-pitched screams pierced the air so sharply that glass would have shattered had there been any around. "Not to worry, you're in good hands. Once we put you inside our unit, we'll get you all taken care of," I told the woman. My words of comfort likely fell on deaf ears. Her focus was the sensational pain coming from her burning left leg. "It feels like it's on fire! It feels like it's on fire right now!" The woman said referring to her leg. "Pain meds are on the way," I told our patient. "Fentanyl sounds like a good drug", I thought to myself while loading her into the truck. Fentanyl is very strong and short acting. There was absolutely no need to ask the usual, "What's your level of pain on a scale of 1 to 10?" because patients who have veins bulging out of their foreheads and eyeballs that look like they are going to jump out of their face convey a "10" without question. Especially when the mechanism of injury (I.E. boat engine exploding on leg) is legitimate for a patient's agonizing groans. Rummaging through our trauma cabinet, I pulled out our sterile burn dressings. I quickly wrapped her thigh. Jeff started an IV and hung a bag of IV fluids. She needed fluid replacement and pain management — fast. "We need to get the fentanyl drawn up like yesterday," Jeff explained while hooking the fluid tubing into the IV port, but I was already on it. Jeff hadn't realized that I grabbed it out of the medications cabinet and was currently drawing it up because he was looking down at what *he* was doing. This tends to happen from time to time during an emergency. Everyone is so busy fumbling with multiple things that you get tunnel vision every once in a while. Speed is beneficial, but accuracy is a must in the pre-hospital setting. The correct treatment must be given because that can be the difference between a good or bad outcome. I double checked the drug dose, drug, expiration date, etc. and slowly pushed the fentanyl into the woman's vein. Her stats were looking just fine on our monitor.

Her blood pressure was a bit low, but nothing way out of bounds. Besides, Jeff and I had taken care of that with running fluids, it was only a matter of time before her blood pressure would rise well within normal limits now. Shortly after the dosage of fentanyl, our female patient grew quieter. Relieved from the pain, to a degree, she relaxed her shoulders finally and sat back against the cot. She let out a long, drawn out sigh of relief. "What would you say your pain is on a scale of 1 to 10, 10 being the worst pain you've ever felt in your life?" I asked. (Now was a time where this question would be appropriate to see if the drugs palliated her pain). "About a 7 out of 10", she replied, followed by another long sigh. The drugs had taken some of the edge off — that is what mattered. We never expected to completely make every ounce of pain disappear. We more so want to bring our patients to a level they can at least tolerate. The burn patient was brought to the closest burn-capable hospital. Her leg would heal in due time.

The Lord is nigh unto all them that call upon him, to all that call upon him in truth. He will fulfill the desire of them that fear him: he also will hear their cry, and will save them.
Psalm 145:18 – 19

#23

Gravity Will Get You

Paramedic Pointer» *Falls account for a large percentage of EMS responses, believe it or not; therein lies an entrepreneurial opportunity. If you can invent an innovative way to prevent falls then you will become an overnight millionaire!*

Ladders present a great way to reach high places. Firemen use them to perform rescues from windows and get cats out of trees, landscapers use them to cut high up tree limbs and construction workers use them in their field. Ladders are not only used for commercial use though, everyday homeowners often have them for odd jobs. That's exactly what one man used his ladder for — a domestic painting project. All he wanted to accomplish was the painting of the upper walls in his home, but somehow he managed to *fall short* of getting that mission done — literally. His house was two stories high, a very nice looking residence. The moment you stepped foot in the house, nothing but sea blue paint surrounded you, except for the upper walls — they were still white. Two ladders were set up on the same wall about 12 feet from one another. Next to the ladder on the left laid a man lying flat on his back, grimacing in pain. Blood was oozing out of his forehead. Three other men were present who saw the fall happen. "He hit that ledge up there on his way down. He landed on that ledge for a split second and continued to fall down to the ground," a man pointed up to the wall as he explained. "He landed sideways on that ledge up there and rolled off. Since that ledge is about halfway up the wall, it helped to break the long fall into two shorter falls," a second witness added. I sized up the wall to be about 24 feet from the ceiling to the floor. Our patient experienced an approximate 12 foot fall two times. Judging by the quality of his head wound, he didn't bump it on the ledge too hard.

Turning my attention to the patient after a moment of scanning the scene, I saw deformity to his right shoulder. Instantly I grew greatly concerned for his collarbone. For one, he was conscious. We paramedics absolutely love to see a patient who is conscious for starters. "Did he pass out at all when he hit the ground?" I turned and asked the three other men standing in the room. "No, he's maintained consciousness the whole time," one of the guys wearing a green T-shirt said. Two major questions we ask in regards to fall victims who have head injuries is "did they lose consciousness" and "are they on blood thinners?" Anytime the head is jolted with trauma, things such as reduced consciousness or even loss of consciousness can occur. Blood thinners are of concern because blood thinners such as Xeralto or Plavix actually increase bleeding. Jeff pulled out a cervical collar (in layman's terms: neck brace) to put on our patient. The whole idea is that the movement of the spine is immobilized. This way, further injury is difficult to incur in the neck. "Where are you hurting?" I asked the patient. "My whole right side is killing me man, absolutely killing me!" The patient moaned. "We're going to place you on a backboard okay sir, but before we move you around at all, I'm going to initiate an IV and give you some pain medication." Jostling and jolting a patient around is a recipe for disaster in serious trauma calls like this one. It's also a great way to become hated if you so much as attempt to move someone in a traumatic situation without treating their pain first. A fall more than 20 feet is what's considered a "significant MOI" or "significant mechanism of injury" in paramedic protocols. Anytime we have a significant injury on our hands, one can expect pain management. Hip fractures are big on the list for pain treatment before moving the patient.

This guy had pipes for veins, which always brings a smile to a care provider's face. *The bigger the better* reigns true for blood vessels because they are harder to miss. The IV was a breeze. I secured his IV site and drew up the Dilaudid that would soon be delivered. Vital signs revealed no red flags, so all systems were a go, so to speak. Dilaudid, being an extremely strong drug, took a minimal amount of time to kick in. "What's your name sir?" I began to build rapport with the patient as the drug entered his body. "Do you have any medical history? You look pretty young sir," I said. He was a Caucasian man with dirty blonde hair and green eyes. "Nope… No medical history yet, I'm 37 years old and healthy. I'm just injured at the moment," he said in a lighthearted fashion. The Dilaudid was starting to kick in well because he confirmed that his pain became a lot more tolerable. He even began to squirm around, moving his head to look around.

"Take it easy, sir. We've got that c-collar on you so that your neck stays where it is — in a stationary position. Jeff had gone to get a backboard and returned saying, "Alrighty… Are we all ready for liftoff?" "Just about," I replied. "I didn't get your name sir, what was it?" I asked the patient while still on my knees. "Michael," the man said. "I'm Lorenzo, by the way, and this is my partner Jeff. Since you're right side is injured, were going to roll you on to your left side and slide this backboard under you," I explained to him. "Whatever you guys need to do," Michael grimaced. "One…two..three..ROLL!" I chanted. Jeff and I slid the backboard under Michael quickly and rolled him back onto it. The maneuver went smoothly. After strapping him in tightly to the board, we lifted him up to place him on our stretcher. Michael kept his eyes closed as he was rolled out of the house and down the driveway. He appeared to be coping well with that deformed shoulder, not to mention the bump on his forehead. Blood was barely oozing out of the cut he had on the bruise, a light dressing would take care of that — no problem.

Michael was monitored intensely on the way to the trauma center. The shoulder ended up being a confirmed dislocation according to x-rays. Michael also fractured his clavicle (collar bone). An additional dose of Dilaudid brought down the pain down to 5 out of 10 on our pain scale. Unhooking our medical probes off of Michael, I lightly placed my hand on his uninjured shoulder and bid him farewell. "Thank you, gentlemen, thank you for everything," he replied.

Lo, children are an heritage of the Lord: and the fruit of the womb is his reward. As arrows are in the hand of a mighty man; so are children of the youth. Happy is the man that hath his quiver full of them: they shall not be ashamed, but they shall speak with the enemies in the gate. **Psalm 127:3 – 5**

#24

Not One, But Dos

Paramedic Pointer» *God considers the number 40 to be significant for testing and change. How interesting, then, that the total time a pregnancy lasts happens to be 40 weeks from conception (first day of last menstrual cycle) to birth.*

My soothing hibernation got interrupted by the insanely sharp sounds of the station 16 notification bells. I can't stress enough how much it felt like an assault on one's ears whenever a call came through at station 16. It happened around 2:30 AM – 3 AM, somewhere within that time span. Long days filled with many calls tax a paramedic's body physically. Report writing, critical thinking and situational awareness contribute to the taxing of the paramedics *mind*. Strenuous shifts translate to a constant beating— blow after blow— a paramedic can get worn down from fatigue.

Today was one of those strenuous shifts. Everything under the sun had happened this shift, it seemed. Everything bad that could happen in the streets *did* happen. Every person whose immune system was weak got even weaker. For these reasons, I fell deep into a coma when finally receiving some downtime. I needed a power nap from all of the relentless abuse delivered to me earlier that day. So out of a deep, deep slumber I was summoned. Just as quickly as I fell into the sleep did I awake from it with the help of those dandy notification tones. Tonight, or this particular morning, I should say, was a morning that would signify a milestone in my personal career. My jumpsuit sat at my bedside. It was rolled down in such a way so that I could step into it and easily pull it up over my body. The jumpsuit had a convenient zipper that ran from the pelvic region all the way up to the collar. My paramedic hat rested on the nightstand right next to my station bed, which I snatched up and slapped onto my head.

Jeff had already jumped in the driver seat, having already started the engine. He began revving up the engine as I opened the passenger door to the flashing ambulance. Jeff, being a true night owl, was psyched about the task set out for us. I was still unaware of what lied before us because the dispatcher's voice sounded like garbled static to my ears when I was waking up. The computer screen showed that we were responding to a pregnant female. Scrolling down the screen revealed, further down, that we didn't have time to waste. The words I saw from the computer screen's call notes read, "Imminent delivery". Suddenly I took a large gulp — the kind of gulp not only the person gulping can hear, but anyone within 5 feet can here too. "We've got to get there fast," Jeff stated with a look of ambition all over his face. He released the airbrake, looked both ways briefly, and plunged into the street for an urgent response.

Few vehicles were on the road, leaving minimal obstructions to swerve through. On the way to the location, it began to rain moderately. Jeff slowed down about 10 mph to avoid hydroplaning. A huge ambulance spinning out of control does no one any good. If anything, it would potentially create more patients and cause an unnecessary burden on other ambulances to bear. It took us approximately four minutes to reach our designated location. Through our swiping windshield wipers I spotted the numbers on a duplex-style establishment that matched our notes. Jeff mashed the brakes to halt, keying up the mobile mic to say, "Medic 16 has arrived on scene". We both turned to the glove rack, which was mounted in between the two of us in the ambulance, grabbing our purple medical gloves.

Next we scrambled to the rear of the truck. Swinging the rear doors open, I leaped inside to grab the obstetrical kit for deliveries. "Let's get inside and see what we're dealing with," Jeff said to me. On the couch laid a young Hispanic woman with an umbilical cord running from her vagina. Connected to her umbilical cord was a newborn baby (already delivered) on a towel. The baby was silent for the most part, making soft noises here and there. I opened up the obstetrics package and grabbed the scalpel. "Be careful not to cut the baby," Jeff cautiously warned me. "I'm going to cut upward so that I'm cutting away from the newborn," I replied to Jeff. Jeff clamped the umbilical cord in two spots about 3 inches apart from one another, leaving the middle as my "sweet spot" to sever. I carefully took the scalpel — blade facing up — and gently rocked back and forth in an upward motion. SNAP! — The umbilical cord broke apart. That scalpel was so sharp that it didn't take much effort at all to cut the cord. To keep the baby warm, we wrapped him in a small blanket, placing a cap on his head.

Back in school, my paramedic instructor would say, "the day will come for some of you when you will need to wrap a newborn up in a blanket properly! So today, I'm going to show you all how to make baby burritos!" Baby burritos were the name given to a newborn baby in a blanket because of the technique one is supposed to wrap the blanketed baby with. Further, newborns are not much larger than a burrito in size! There was a man on scene standing behind the mother. Mommy was laying long ways on a couch, and who I assume to have been the father, stood to the right of the couch, just behind mommy's head. "That was easy," I said to myself. How easier could it have possibly been? All we had to do was cut a cord and wrap a baby up. Turns out, I celebrated prematurely. Darn. Stepping over to daddy, who Jeff had handed the newborn baby to already, I congratulated him with a light pat on the back. "You're a father now, sir," I said with a big smile. "Congratulations!" Daddy shot me back a smile and murmured, "Ehhh....gracias!"

Both parents were Hispanic. Neither of them spoke any English. It didn't seem to be an issue since the baby was already here. Not much instruction or communication absolutely had to go on, per se, at this point. But things took a sudden turn — something unexpected. Jeff and I were sort of basking in the beauty of creation, along with the parents, when suddenly the mood all changed. Daddy's smile faded slowly, but not fading into an angry or sad look. His face simply turned neutral. Daddy, cradling the newborn in one arm, held up two fingers with his free hand. "Ehhh… Dos," uttered the father, pointing to the Hispanic mother laid out on the sofa. "Dos babies??" I questioned him, pointing to the newborn while holding up the number "two" with my other hand. "Si…Si" daddy nodded his head up and down. Jeff and I took about a total of one second to let the information sink in. "Eeeeeyyyeeaaahhh…. Let's get going," Jeff said to me while already snatching up our medical bags. "I'll run our bags out to the truck and be back to help load mommy up," I told Jeff as I took them out of his hands. The rain had picked up, I noticed, when making that quick run. The purpose behind making a quick run was because we couldn't fit all of our equipment on the stretcher along with the patient. We would have had to carry the bags *and* try to steer the stretcher simultaneously. Doing that is a huge no-no. Two hands on the stretcher is the safest way to operate, especially when there's a patient on it!

Returning from my quick sprint to the ambulance, we wasted no time in placing mommy on our cot. Daddy was motioned, via hand gestures, to hold the delivered baby in his arms and ride with us—he understood.

Rolling across their yard was bumpy. The yard was uncut and unleveled. Through the rain we moved diligently across the front lawn, being careful to keep the cot balanced. A common fear of paramedics is to drop a patient, or God forbid, allow a bad angle of terrain to tip the stretcher over with someone on it. Above all, it's a danger to the patient. After that come lawsuits, stressful hang-ups and very likely, the loss of one's job. There's pretty much zero tolerance for injuring a patient.

Successfully making it through the yard brought us to the rear of the ambulance. Jeff on one side of the cot and myself on the opposite side, our team effort to load mommy inside our truck was absolutely the fastest ever. "Emergency transport…keep it nice and slow," Jeff said to me with caution. *Emergency transport* meant that we would transport using lights and sirens. Another term we use to refer to this transport urgency is *running hot*. Jeff and I both knew that we only had a few minutes before a second baby would be here. We made the decision to leave instead of deliver at her house because the hospital was only five minutes away, three or four turns and we'd be in the ER parking lot. It was a nice, easy ride. Virtually no cars were out on the road due to it being 3:45 AM or so.

Reaching the hospital grounds marked a turning point. "Wherever you're at, stop the truck and jump back here — I need help!" Jeff frantically shouted from the back of the ambulance. Our trucks front tires had literally just made contact with what was considered hospital property. I pulled over to the nearest curb and raced to the back to help Jeff deliver. An ER paramedic who must have been just coming in or taking a break was passing nearby. "Hey you! Grab a few extra hands, we've got a mother crowning back here (crowning is when a newborn's head is showing from the vagina)!" I yelled to him. Jeff had an innumerable amount of white towels out to help catch blood. He also had a few placed under the mother's hips. "Ahhhhh…..AHHHHHHHH!!!!" The high-pitched screams of the mother filled our truck. Five medical personnel showed up, including the paramedic I asked to retrieve them. There were three female nurses and two ER medics, to be exact. Everyone gloved up and jumped in to help facilitate delivery.

My God, was it a bloody mess in the back of that ambulance. Never have I seen so much blood at one time. "PUUUSSSHHHH!" Coached a female nurse. "BREATHE… NOW PUSH!!" She continuously directed the mother. PLOP! —Out came the baby. After the head and shoulders came out, the second half of the baby's body spit out in an instant. It was as if he was being regurgitated. The beautiful newborn boy began crying. A crying baby is desired because it means that his or her airway is open. Creation was a beauty to behold —a *bittersweet* one at that. All of the stress from giving birth caused a flare-up around mommy's mouth that resembled herpes. Upon transferring care to the receiving ER nurse, a familiar look came over the nurse's face. "Oh wow… *She's* back again," the nurse stated. "This isn't her first rodeo, not by a longshot," she continued. "This 24-year-old mother is a heroin addict and prostitute. She also has a history of herpes. That's what all *that* is around her mouth," the nurse said while waving an open hand around her own mouth. (These statements were made beyond the ears of our patient, by the way).

"Yeah, it's such a shame that people like this squander their gift of being able to conceive. My sister can't even have children!" The nurse grew impatient, shaking her head in dismay. I empathized with the nurse for a few moments, soon bidding her a farewell.

"What on earth was that?!" Jeff asked me in shock as we paced the hospital hall. "You just never know what awaits you around the corner," I replied. "She was a total disaster! I was hoping her blood wouldn't splash me in the eye; you could tell she had an STD from a mile away!" Jeff said. We exited the labor and delivery department, heading back to our ambulance. There was a mess waiting on us to be cleaned up.

The fear of the Lord is to hate evil: pride, and arrogancy, and the evil way, and the froward mouth, do I hate. **Proverbs 8:13**

#25

Drug-Induced Powerhouse

Paramedic Pointer» *Pinpoint pupils are a telltale sign of narcotic use.*

It's not the size of the dog that's in the fight— it's the size of the fight that's in the dog. This age-old saying reigned true for a young woman who took drugs and ended up unconscious. She was sprawled out on the concrete parking lot of an EMS station. The unit assigned to that EMS station was out on call. Naturally, the responsibility fell on the closest unit available, which happened to be Jeff and me. We were on our way back from dropping a patient off at the ER when the call was given to us.

"We have a female patient — age unknown — unconscious…" Our dispatch reported candidly. Cruising down the street towards what we thought would be our home station; this notification prompted Jeff to make a sharp turn down an alley, stopping for just a few seconds to look at the computer map. It's never a good outcome when one tries to zoom to an unfamiliar area. Every now and again a newbie flicks the emergency lights on and mashes the gas pedal before the dispatcher even gets the address out of their mouth completely. That reaction is probably one of adrenaline, eagerness or plain old nervousness. No matter the reason, I love to hear the response when I sit back for a moment and ask, "where we going?" That's when that *scattered brain* effect quickly *un-scatters* and the newbie pumps the brakes because they realize that they haven't even a clue yet.

Be no mistake, we knew where our fellow EMS station was located without mapping, but as a rule, we always double checked our location because sometimes locations can be misquoted, mistyped or change while en route. Continuing towards our given location, it turned out to be about three minutes before we rolled up on the downed female. Our responding fire truck arrived simultaneously. Out of the fire truck stepped three firemen ready to intervene. Jeff and I unloaded our stretcher in a hurry, fully stocked with our equipment. Her respirations were extremely slow; one could barely see her chest rise and fall. I handed the bag valve mask (breathing delivery device) to the closest fireman standing near me so that I could fish out my IV supplies. It didn't take but one or two seconds, it was only a matter of unzipping the top compartment of our blue medical bag. Our IV box sat on top of everything for easy access. The IV box was clear/see-through and held multiple needles, tourniquets, syringes, alcohol prep pads, etc. Unclicking this clear IV kit marked the sound of business needing to be handled. CLICK-CLICK!!—I rounded up my IV equipment and began the process. My IV turned out to be successful. A fireman checked the woman's pupils and said, "These eyes are pinpoint!" He was referring to her eyes so that everyone on scene would comprehend the likelihood of her having overdosed on a narcotic.

In the County of Manatee, here in Florida, heroin is the All-Star narcotic — everyone seems to have some. I drew up my Narcan (narcotic antidote drug) from its box and pushed it through my established IV access point. Thankfully, the typical *reawakening* of our downed patient occurred — but let's just say she was a tad bit more than simply *awake*. It wasn't as if a slow moving mummy had been awoken from its tomb — more like a Bengal tiger who needed an anger management class. Just when the medication kicked in, our patient kicked in the stomach of the fireman located just beyond her legs. This particular fireman drew the short straw. Five of us were knelt down around this young female as she returned to consciousness kicking and screaming her brains out. About half the time, it seems, when you bring an overdose patient back from unconsciousness, they are absolutely perturbed. What has happened in returning to a conscious state is their high has been blown. The high they spend their money on trying earnestly to achieve. For this reason, they are ridiculously pissed and want to fight any and every one — because in the patient's eyes, everyone needs to pay for their actions. Everyone, in this particular moment deserves severe punishment. Physical punishment — a *beat down* to be specific. You think five men versus one female— a small one at that— would be no contest. Not so. Not so at all when you throw drugs in the mix of things. A driver's license fell out of her back pocket while she was thrashing around recklessly. The nearest fireman speedily snagged her card and announced, "Her name is Caitlin". "Calm down Caitlin, we're here to help you!" Jeff scolded her. SLAP!!—Caitlin, with no hesitation, cocked back her hand and smacked Jeff across his face with full force. You should've seen that look Jeff had on his face. Time stood completely still that moment. Jeff wanted to maul the woman — it was written all over his temperamental facial expression. I was elated to see that he kept a leveled head (meaning no physical retaliation).

"All right Caitlin, that's it! I've had it with you!" Jeff scolded. All three of the on scene firemen were in the process of restraining Caitlin with what we call *soft restraints*. They were tying Caitlin to the stretcher, each extremity individually. Behind her, I was drawing up a medication called haloperidol (an antipsychotic). Handing the drawn up medication to Jeff, he quickly punctured her outside shoulder tissue, also known as the deltoid muscle. It wasn't much longer that Caitlin continued to fuss and fight. The handy haloperidol did its job well. The fight was officially over. Her respirations were back up to normal. Caitlin, now stable and completely manageable, had fallen fast asleep.

Expediting her transport became top priority, Jeff raced to the driver seat and to the hospital we fled. Time was of the essence because that haloperidol would wear off sooner or later — drugs don't last forever. Also, crazy acting females are a situation male medics try to steer clear of as much as possible. All it takes is a bipolar, psychotic or flat out lying female to say one of us touched her inappropriately. Only negativity ensues an individual from that point until the accusation is resolved. And without witnesses, it can be a tough situation to deal with. I can't speak for all ambulance agencies, but generally speaking, ambulance trucks are not equipped with surveillance cameras. Caitlin stayed asleep until it was time for her to be transferred. "She's a bit of a wild child," I warned the ER nurse. My receiving nurse paged security. "If you keep miss Caitlin restrained, you'll be happy you did". The nurse signed my report and began to prepare for the worst.

For the eyes of the Lord run to and fro throughout the whole earth, to shew himself strong on the behalf of them whose heart is perfect toward Him. Herein thou hast done foolishly: therefore from henceforth thou shalt have wars. **2 Chronicles 16:9**

#26

I'm Not Crazy!

Paramedic Pointer» The textbook blood pressure considered to be normal is 120/80 mmHg. Blood pressures are measured in millimeters of mercury. The blood pressure cuff's true name is "sphygmomanometer".

Assaults are such a common occurrence in the world of EMS that a paramedic can tend to downplay assaults, to be honest. I can't tell you how many times an assault came in through our dispatch and we show up to find that the victim of the assault has a scraped knee from being pushed down. By no means am I saying that a scraped knee doesn't hurt — but a frantic call to 911 for it? Even as a guy who always gives the benefit of the doubt, come on, give me a break. A discipline we paramedics have to employ is to not get comfortable in making assumptions based off of what *typically* happens.

Jeff and I received a call for an assault that was leaps and bounds beyond a scraped knee. The call was located at a mental counseling office. Midday, in the pinnacle of the sun's ferocious heat, Jeff and I stepped off of the ambulance with a belly full of lunch. We had only been directly across the street trying to scarf down a meal from Wawa. Outside of the office stood a Caucasian woman in business attire. Greeting us in a concerned manner, she began, "Your patient is inside, to the left, sitting down with an ice pack on her eye… It's swollen shut". "Is the person who assaulted her still on scene?" I asked the woman. "No… It was her son who beat her up. He jumped on her in the parking lot and stole her car… he took off," she finished. Jeff and I briskly continued into the mental health office. A stocky black woman sat crying in a chair with her head tilted upward. Tears ran down her plump cheeks as she sniffled every few seconds. "Hello Miss, I'm Lorenzo and this is my partner Jeff," I introduced us both. "Could you explain to me exactly what happened today?" I said. Lifting up the ice pack she had resting on her right eye revealed a nasty bruise. Both bottom and top of her right eye was swollen — her right eye was completely closed. "Umm…" She began, trying to gain a hold of her composure. "I came here with my son… I was trying to get him help by professionals… He's always sitting around smiling all day long and looking at the walls. He's 26 years old now, so I made him move out of my house. He's been back lately… sneaking into my garage and sleeping in there. So I allowed him to stay with me until I could get an appointment made for him to be seen."

When we were in the parking lot, he turned to me and screamed, "I'M NOT CRAZY". That's when he body slammed me and started punching me in the face!" The stocky woman explained. She scooted down in her chair at that point and continued to cry. "Help is here now, Miss," I told her sincerely. I broke out my stethoscope and blood pressure cuff to obtain a manual blood pressure on her left arm. Her pulse felt strong and her blood pressure was a bit high. "Did you lose consciousness at all when your son slammed you on the parking lot pavement?" I asked. "Do you mean like blackout?" She questioned. "Yes, that's exactly what I mean," I replied. "I think I did blackout for about five seconds when he kept punching me over and over," she cried. "Why would he do this to me? I'm his mother! I'm the one who took care of him for all of these years!" She blurted out while continuing to drench her round cheeks in tears. "What is your name?" I asked the sobbing woman. "Tara… My name is Tara," she said through short sniffles. "Let's try to stand and pivot onto my stretcher so that we can give you something for that pain inside my truck," I encouraged her. She slowly stood up from her chair and plopped down onto the cot. Tara swung her legs up onto the cot as well, prompting Jeff and I to begin buckling her in safely. Everyone in the waiting room stopped what they were doing to spectate. Two women who were chatting stopped talking to each other. A few people entertaining themselves on their phones had paused their games. It was a quiet exit out of the office as everyone gazed at Tara's atrocious right eye trauma. Police were in the parking lot discussing what happened with a witness.

Once inside the truck, we gave Tara a fresh ice pack — the ice given to her by the inside office personnel had melted for the most part. Tara maintained her head tilted upward, staring at the ceiling of the ambulance in awe. She was probably *seeing stars* as they say; her head was without a doubt, severely rattled. Jeff and I decided to go with a lighter pain medication on this call, not the usual narcotic pain meds. The drug we used is called Toradol. It's a nonsteroidal anti-inflammatory drug. I administered 30 mg of Toradol through my established IV. Facial pain, especially at the level of the skin (bruising) is not quite a sufficient reason to administer pain medication at the narcotic level. Toradol has the effect ibuprofen has, they are both the same class of drug, but Toradol works faster because the route it's administered to a person in is quicker. Since Toradol directly enters the bloodstream by way of IV, it is faster acting than an ibuprofen pill (usually about 20 – 30 minutes to kick in). "What is your pain right now?" I asked Tara, to obtain a baseline. "OH!! ABOUT A 10 OUT OF 10!!!!" She cried. I gave her the Toradol after obtaining her pain scale. Now it was a matter of allowing the drug to take effect. Tara's blood pressure was a bit high, but this was the only outstanding concern. She had no other injuries upon assessment. En route to the hospital, Tara was monitored closely. To my satisfaction, she remained in a stable condition very well.

A policewoman met us at the ER. "Would you like to press charges on your son?" The police woman asked intently. "YES, ABSOLUTELY!!" Cried Tara, who turned out to be 52 years old. "I want to press charges in full!" She continued. Somewhere out in the streets roamed Tara's son. He had yet to be found, but you can believe that the police force was on the case like bloodhounds.

The Lord shall open up unto thee his good treasure, the heaven to give the rain unto thy land in his season, and to bless all the work of thine hand: and thou shalt lend unto many nations, and thou shalt not borrow. **Deuteronomy 28:12**

#27

When Stealing Dad's Car Goes Wrong

Paramedic Pointer» *Direct pressure with a gloved hand, towel, trauma dressing or gauze can stop venous bleeding (slow, oozing flow). Arterial bleeding (squirting blood) will likely need a tourniquet placed above the wounded site to cease bleeding adequately.*

I think it's safe to say we've all thought about taking our parents' car for a spin in our adolescence; for some, maybe even earlier than that. Some of us simply went ahead and *did it*. I can remember taking my mother's car out for a joy ride with my older sister growing up. Of course my brother, who couldn't keep his mouth shut if the world depended on it, let the cat out of the bag. I can also remember taking my uncle's Ford expedition out for a cruise in the middle of the night with my favorite cousin. Both of these occasions were lots of fun. It made me feel cool, dangerous and dare devilish. Very few times did I actually get caught joyriding with my parents' vehicle or my uncle's Ford expedition. I cannot recall how many times to be exact — it was definitely either once or twice. What I can recall perfectly was the number of times I was hurt or in any danger from joyriding — zero. I thank God for keeping such a young, ignorant knucklehead like myself safe and sound; it truly was and is a blessing. Not every adolescent can be so lucky — it's just the way things are in the world — nothing is perfect.

This is the story of two young teenage boys who had a need for speed that quickly turned into a need for an ambulance. There's an affluent community called Snell Isle that Jeff and I responded to, this is where the mishap took place. Snell Isle stood apart from most neighborhoods I've responded to. Every resident kept a fresh looking yard. Great quality grass, impressive shrubbery, and beautiful palm trees contributed to the eye-pleasing landscape. Smack dab in the middle of this particular community was a huge circle with grass in the center. What I'm describing is often referred to as a *roundabout*. Skid marks from the tires decorated the street encircling this grassy roundabout. Off to the right was a jet black Camaro wrapped around a palm tree — it's a wonder how the Camaro didn't slice evenly in half. Moving closer to the wreckage as Jeff and I hopped out of the truck revealed that the passenger — a young Caucasian male— was thrown out onto the pavement. He laid there, his back to the ground, with a slow flow of blood trickling down the corner of his mouth. Night time made visibility a temporary problem; it was approximately midnight in a poorly lit segment of the neighborhood streets.

CLICK!—Jeff pressed the button on his flashlight. Scanning the boy's body from head to toe, a pool of blood came into view when Jeff shined the LED flashlight on his upper body. I knelt down to examine our first patient. The young man had no pulse. He also had a gash in the back of his head that exposed both skull and brain matter. "He's DOA (dead on arrival)," I announced. Just ahead was the blacked out Camaro, accompanied by smoke puffing out of the hood. I saw a young man leaned forward on the steering wheel with blood cascading down his head in three small streams — they were traveling from a laceration on his forehead. The airbag in the steering wheel had clearly deployed. The white airbag drooped down from the steering wheel due to it being deflated at the time. Leaning down into the driver's side door, I checked the young boy's pulse at his neck. "THIS PATIENT HAS A PULSE!!" I yelled to Jeff. Other than the laceration on the patient's forehead, he didn't appear to have further injury elsewhere. I could tell by the weakness of his pulse that his blood pressure was very low.

A fireman walked up to us carrying a backboard to put our patient on. "Were going to place it under his butt and have another person manage his upper body while we move him onto the board. We're taking him out feet first!" I declared. Before the whole sentence came out of my mouth, the same fireman who brought the backboard in such timely fashion positioned his self perfectly in the passenger seat. "Ready! One... Two... Three... Move!" I counted off, before myself, Jeff and the fireman placed our patient on the backboard to be carried over to the cot. His respirations were dangerously low. All three of us (Jeff, myself and the fireman) pushed the stretcher as fast as we could without jeopardizing our patient's safety. Jeff was at the foot, I was at the head, and the fireman stabilized the side of the stretcher as we made haste to the ambulance. "Grab a bag valve mask!" I urged the fireman. He flung the airway cabinet open, ripped open the device packaging and tossed it over to me. It was paramount to establish control over the patient's airway. Jeff began squeezing breaths into the patient; I was preparing the intubation equipment. I was just seconds away from placing a tube down our patient's airway — the optimal way to breathe for a patient.

"Okay I'm ready Jeff," I told him. Jeff removed the bag valve mask from our patient's mouth and I performed the process of intubation. Jeff confirmed it to be successful by listening over the lungs with his stethoscope. "You're in!" Jeff said with satisfaction. "Do you all want me to ride along?" The fireman questioned. "I think we can handle it," Jeff said with confidence. I didn't object. Out jumped the fireman, exiting through the rear ambulance doors. I maintained our patient's airway; Jeff started a large-bore IV in the patient's forearm. The larger (diameter) the IV is, the more fluid that can be delivered. Our patient needed lots of fluid; the young Caucasian male had lost consciousness upon crashing into that pessimistic palm tree. He was still alive though, much better than his friend who did not make it.

During transport to the ER, our fluids proved to be effective, raising his low blood pressure back up to normal limits. We made sure his intubation tube stayed securely fastened in place. Delivering the young boy to the ER safely, we reported that the other young male was dead on arrival; this brought on a dismal moment of silence. Chance of survival looked good for the unconscious patient, but only time would tell of his functionality once completely conscious again. Two young boys just going out for a joyride with daddy's car turned into one life lost. They were so caught in the moment that the patient who got thrown out of the vehicle forgot about wearing a seatbelt. This night will not be forgotten. Not by Jeff. Not by myself. And certainly not by either of the young boy's parents. Be safe out there.

Be ye strong therefore, and let not your hands be weak: for your work shall be rewarded. **2 Chronicles 15:7**

#28

Orange Juice and a Heart Attack

Paramedic Pointer» *The human heart can pump 5-7 liters of blood per minute, that's 2,000 gallons per day.*

Bradenton, Florida is the home of one Tropicana juice factory. If you drive around with your windows down, one can smell the aroma of oranges throughout the air. I'm told that the scent radiating from the factory is from orange peels being burnt. It makes sense. After all, they've got to do something to get rid of all those leftover peels. I always thought it'd be cool to go inside to see how they produced orange juice so fast. Witnessing the process would be something neat, it seemed. Well, I got my chance to take a tour; only under circumstances I would rather not have been the cause. "Woman down at Tropicana juice factory" is what Jeff and I's call notes read. Further down the computer screen, it read, "Employee not alert". When we stepped foot inside the factory, I was overwhelmed by all the machinery spinning, sliding and shifting. From the moment we got in the factory, there were conveyor belts on all four levels carrying ungodly amounts of oranges. There was a handy security guard who took us to the stairwell; our patient was located on the fourth floor.

Jeff took one bag in his hand, our laptop in the other. I carried our other two bags. Pacing up the metal steps, I occasionally scanned the factory to observe my loud surroundings. It wasn't only the gigantic machinery moving about that was intimidating, but the combination of loud noise as well. Our stairwell allowed one to get off at every level. On the third level, we had to cut across pretty much the entire factory to a new set of steps— It felt like such a long journey. I'm telling you, without fail, Jeff and I always get patients who are the absolute furthest away from the entrance of an establishment. It works like a charm. With nursing home facilities, with grocery stores, with schools, etc. — It is always the last room, row, column or aisle.

Finally making it up to the fourth floor, a woman came into our view. She was slouched down in a chair positioned up against a conveyor belt. The chair had a swivel so that the chair could spin a half circle's range. Our female patient was sweating profusely. She was drenched from head to toe. Thankfully, the woman had a pulse. She was an older black woman, approximately 55 years old or so. Wrapping a blood pressure cuff around her upper arm, I quickly pumped the cuff up and listened intently. It was an average blood pressure, but on the lower end of a normal range. I then snatched out some 4 x 4 gauze to wipe down the woman's diaphoretic (sweaty) chest. To assess her heart, stickers needed to be placed on her chest. This would allow us to take a picture of her heart with our cardiac monitor. 20 seconds later, our snapshot came back. To a person not medically trained this *snapshot* would look like a bunch of squiggly lines. "SHE'S HAVING A HEART ATTACK!" I announced. A fireman brought up a piece of equipment called a stair chair, made for getting patients down staircases. Stretchers just aren't designed for stairs. "If you lift from her left side (under her armpit), I'll lift her up from her right side," I told the fireman. Jeff prepared the stair chair by unbuckling its seatbelts and holding it firmly in place. Gently lowering the black woman onto the chair, we maneuvered her limp body so that we could fasten the top seatbelt under her arms. There's a footstool that flips out on the bottom of the stair chair for patients to put their feet on — we made proper use of this.

Traveling back down to floor one was a bit quicker, yet much louder. Each level was made of metal flooring with holes in it, making for a very metallic vibration as our stair chair wheels rolled across it. Hundreds of oranges tumbled down and across the multiple conveyor belts simultaneously — this was orange juice heaven. Though her body was limp and lifeless, she was packaged tightly with the seatbelt straps — she wasn't going anywhere, as bumpy as the ride in the stair chair was. A decline awaited us, spanning from the factory doors to the ambulance. Two workers taking a smoke break outside stopped their conversation and watched in silence as we rolled by to the truck. Jeff snatched some oxygen tubing out of the airway cabinet and chucked it at me. I connected it to our oxygen tank and carefully placed the oxygen cannula's prongs in her nostrils. An important intervention to make with cardiac patients, specifically heart attacks, is oxygen administration. Your heart has an oxygen demand, and even more so during heart attacks.

"Medic 16 to the ER... I've got a patient having a heart attack, not alert... This will be a priority one transport," Jeff reported on the mobile mic. By now it was time to rock and roll. Flicking on the ambulance flashers, I then flipped the sirens switch, approaching the factory's security gate — because just outside these gates lied an intersection. The passing traffic would need to see and hear me in the truck so that they would stop. Intersections are the craziest parts of traffic for an ambulance. People listening to music at the highest volumes are not thinking about having to stop for an emergency when it's a green light. So I made lots of noise, mashing the offensively loud air horn and changing the siren's tone patterns. When all cars came to a complete stop, I drove out to the center of the vast intersection and made a right hand turn. It wasn't long before we arrived at the ER—approximately six minutes or so.

"The ER Doc asked us to take her straight up to the Cardiac Cath Lab," Jeff said. Our patient was completely out of it, so to speak. Her head was limp, hanging in a downward angle. It looked like how a person who nods off into a deep sleep does when sitting upright. Her bottom lip hung down a bit, her mouth slightly open. Making a sharp left hand turn into the cardiac Cath Lab brought into focus two doctors. I told them all what happened and we transferred care. Jeff and I began to clean up, changing our stretcher's sheets. Later that day, we found out that our patient would need a few stents placed. Stents are medical solutions designed to keep blood vessels in your heart open. The leading cause of a heart attack is what's called a thrombus, or *obstruction* of vessel(s) in the heart, in other words. This obstruction (blood clot) impedes blood flow, giving one a heart attack.

On the positive side, our patient would be okay. Had we not been there when we were, her outcome may have been different. But as far as our duty goes as professional paramedics, timely responses and positive outcomes are what we strive for, and today punctuality paid off.

And he shall be like a tree planted by the rivers of water, that bringeth forth his fruit in his season; his leaf also shall not wither; and whatsoever he doeth shall prosper. **Psalm 1:3**

#29

Black Out on a Boat Deck

Paramedic Pointer» *Fainting, or syncope (medical term), is the temporary decrease of perfusion to the brain.*

It always intrigued me to hear of people living on boats. A fellow named Joe experienced difficulties when getting off of his. He was stepping off of his personal yacht when suddenly he slipped and fell. Or was it the event of *passing out* that caused him to fall on the dock that happened to be wet? Evening time came upon my partner Jeff and I quickly this shift. Stingrays decided to sting a few beach bums on this particular day, so Jeff and I were already out on the coast taking care of that. There's nothing to stingray stings, really. A bucket of hot water to neutralize the stingray's toxins will suffice. Whatever you do, don't treat it like a bruise and put an ice pack on it! The goal is to neutralize the toxins, and it will in turn, ease the swelling.

Before we could get on to the causeway to exit the beach, a call came in that Jeff and I were the closest unit to. Instead of heading back to the main lands, we hung a hard right, continuing down the beach's coast line to handle a syncopal episode (fainting). It didn't take any more than four minutes to reach the location. *Mooring Field* is a term used here in Florida to refer to a place where multiple boats are secured or anchored. Think of a mooring field as a parking garage, only for boats, not cars. And instead of land, replace that with water. This is where our patient lived. His yacht was halfway down a long boat dock located behind a big factory of some sort. The only land directly to the left of this anonymous factory was a thin strip of concrete just wide enough for our stretcher to fit on. And, to the left of the concrete strip was ocean water. There were potholes and hex headed screws protruding upward from this narrow slab as well. It made traveling back towards the long boat dock a bit nerve racking, what with the constant jostling and jolting of the stretcher as we pushed along the side of the factory.

"This is going to be an interesting trek back to our ambulance once we have our patient," Jeff joked with an uneasy chuckle. "If he tips over into the water, I'm blaming you," I pointed at Jeff with one hand while pushing the cot with my other. Safely surviving the narrow slab of concrete, we made a 90° right turn to approach the long boat dock, which was made of sturdy wood. Our patient could be seen off in the distance, about 40 yards out. He was lying flat on his back, arms and legs stretched out wide. Based off of his completely limp appearance, you would have thought his tongue was even hanging out of his mouth like on some dramatic cartoon clip. Loose coins were strewn about all around the man lying flat on his back. He smelled of alcohol. He wore khaki cargo shorts and a button up Hawaiian shirt that wasn't buttoned up. His hairy chest and pop belly rested out in the open. The middle-aged man grimaced, apperaing to be disoriented. Also, his eyes were squinted as if his vision was blurred. "How did you end up on the ground sir?" I asked the downed patient. "I umm… I uhh…" He struggled to collect his thoughts enough to deliver a sensible response. Another yacht owner came out of his boat that was anchored about 10 yards away. "I saw what happened… I saw the whole thing. This man was walking and suddenly stopped. He stood still for only a moment… And then he just collapsed; he fell down as if his life force was sucked right out of him! It was like watching an inflated balloon lose all of its air in two seconds flat," the other yacht owner stated. "Sounds to me like the man fainted," I turned and told Jeff. "Although, he does smell of alcohol, so he might have fallen down because he had too much to drink," I rationalized.

I knelt down right beside our discombobulated patient and took his blood pressure. It was considerably low. His heart was a bit faster than normal limits.

"What's the last thing you remember Sir?" I asked the patient. "…Uhh… all I remember was walking and then everything turned black… I blacked out!" The patient said nervously. "How much have you had to drink today sir?" I questioned. "Two drinks, that's all," he responded. "Has this ever happened to you before — blacking out like this?" I inquired. "Yes, one time that I can recall… It happened about three years ago."

Our next move was to set up an IV to regain his fallen blood pressure to a normal range. Seagulls swooped down around the dock on which we managed our patient, there were so many of them. "Lay still and don't speak for about 20 seconds, sir," I instructed our patient. I had just got done placing the stickers, or electrodes, as we call them, to run a 12 lead EKG. A 12 lead EKG is a picture of a person's heart. It allows paramedics to evaluate important cardiac imbalances such as heart attacks. When the 12 lead EKG completed its cycle, we leaned our patient up into a sitting position. "We're going to help you up, but we're going to need you to help us out by using your legs," I told the patient. "Okay, I think I can do that," he replied. Jeff and I grabbed under each of his arms and lifted upward in sync, placing him on our stretcher. Hanging our IV fluids proved to be beneficial. Out of a 1000 mL bag of IV fluids, our patient drained almost half of our bag in a blink. This revealed his much needed beckon for fluid intervention.

The 12 lead EKG came back with no red flag — our printout was unremarkable. After assessing vital signs once more, we secured all stretcher seatbelts tightly and began our way back to the ambulance for transport. It was a noisier, and not to mention, bumpier trip back down the long boat dock with the patient now on our stretcher. We took the thin slab of concrete I mentioned before extremely slow. It was pretty ridiculous how narrow that strip was, if I wasn't on an emergency call, I would have phoned in a service request to have it widened for public safety right then and there. "I'm feeling nauseous," our patient groaned. Jeff handed him an emesis bag to hold just in case he vomited. With his blood pressure back up to a normal range at this time, general supportive care and monitoring appeared to be all that he needed. Placing an oxygen cannula in his nose, I then heard Jeff rev up the ambulance engine — it was time to get going to the ER.

The way of the slothful man is as an hedge of thorns: but the way of the righteous is made plain. **Proverbs 15:19**

#30

Sleeping In Fecal Matter

Paramedic Pointer» A normal heart rate is 60-100 beats per minute. If an individual is in great physical shape, it may be naturally lower at rest. Alternately, if one is excited or exerting themselves (such as exercising), it is not abnormal to have higher heart rates.

There's a medical term used to define the loss of urinary and bowel control. The term is called *incontinence*. Incontinence is often associated with seizure patients. When seizure patients undergo a seizure, their involuntary convulsions (shaking) are also accompanied by the loss of control over their bladder/bowels. I wish we could truthfully peg Sherry's incident to be incontinence. Instead, we have to come to the startling acceptance that Sherry's accident was voluntary. Our call dispatch screen generated the emergency code "sick person". This tends to be the code they assign patients with vague complaints such as, "I'm not feeling well" or, "I'm ill". From the moment my partner and I stepped foot into a monstrosity aiming to be a house, an eerie theme of depression inundated our minds. What seemed like 1 million cats were running around everywhere! The rank smell of urine filled the air as if it were taking the place of a lemon scented Lysol freshener. There were no bed frames to be found, only dirty mattresses lying on the floor.

There's nothing wrong with mattresses on the ground, but when they are almost entirely black, one may want to consider getting either a new mattress or bed frame. All in all, the place was a dump. There were four females that occupied the studio apartment. Our patient was located in one corner of the room. She was lying down on a disgustingly dark mattress filled with dirt and grime. All I wanted to do was hold my breath until we got out of there but I needed to communicate with the patient. "What's going on today, miss?" I asked as I knelt down beside her bed. "I'm just not feeling well," she replied. "I couldn't sleep last night. I've peed on myself two times now." "Do you have a history of seizures?" "No, never had one in my life." "Hmm," I thought to myself. "Let's get you onto our cot so that we can further evaluate you inside of our ambulance.

My main concern, once realizing that she was completely stable, was getting out of that apartment before my partner and I suffocated. We wrapped Sherry in white sheets to keep her bodily contents as concealed as we could. The look on her face was one of defeat as we rolled her out to our unit. Upon assessing her from head to toe in the truck, nothing appeared to be wrong with Sherry. "What exactly *is* wrong with you?" I asked in great curiosity. From what I could gather, she called because she wasn't feeling "happy", which is not a medical problem. "I peed on myself two times last night… I also pooped on myself while lying in bed". Taking the statement for what it was worth at face value, I asked, "Why didn't you just get up and use the restroom?" "Oh I'm depressed. I didn't feel like getting out of bed to do anything. I can't find the motivation". What on earth could leave a person depressed so much as to neglect their own wellbeing to this degree? And so I proceeded to find out, "What's got you so depressed Sherry?" Sherry let out a long, drawn out sigh and said, "My mother passed". I can empathize with being depressed over a parent dying— losing loved ones is tough. But the fact that Sherry was content with pooping and peeing her pants over it did not add up. "When did your mother pass away?" I asked.

"She passed away when I was nine years old, never did get over it." Okay hold on. You mean to tell me that someone can actually grieve a loss for that long? That long, meaning 57 years! Sherry was 66 years old! There was no humanly possible way she could have allowed this loss to ail her for 57 years! Immediately I began to assume that Sherry had mental problems, and I say that respectfully. It turns out that she did admit to a history of chronic anxiety and depression, which people do receive medication for. Nonetheless, I can only imagine how emotionally unstable an individual has to be to allow something to fester for that amount of time. Depression is not always an easy thing to overcome for people. Situations I've witnessed seem to resemble that of dominoes — one bad thing happens, triggering another bad thing, so on and so forth. A gentleman we picked up from the Salvation Army had wondered why he was always getting his things stolen. He had his carpentry tools stolen, his clothes stolen, and even his prescribed medication stolen from him!

All he could do was cry about how he was consistently a victim of others. He would say things like, "Why me?" Or "I'm tired of being the victim". It was as if he didn't know he could go and get another job, buy more carpentry tools and fight to get himself back on solid ground. What we have to be careful of as individuals is giving up all hope. This leads to feeling sorry for ourselves instead of fighting to stay afloat. Life is not always a cakewalk. The vast majority of us are not born with everything taken care of already. One man said life is a giant pool of problems and living is *solving* those problems. Wherever you are at this point in your life, please make a conscious effort to never give in, no matter how hard things get for you. It's easy to roll over and waste away! What is truly honored and commendable is the tenacity to rise above the adversity. So my message to you is: don't let anything lay you low; instead, rise above and ascend higher than your setbacks.

My son, forget not my law; but let thine heart keep my commandments: for length of days, and long life, and peace, shall they add to thee. **Proverbs 3:1 – 2**

#31

Status Epilepticus

Paramedic Pointer» A common concern people have for seizure patients is the biting of the tongue while convulsing (shaking). Do not place anything in the mouth of a seizing patient (example: bite block). It could obstruct the airway, which seizing patients do not have control over.

The title of this story refers to an event where multiple seizures happen consecutively without the recovery of consciousness between each seizure. It's a very dangerous phenomenon that is potentially life-threatening. What happens when a person has a seizure is completely involuntary. Though there isn't one key cause of seizures, multiple things can be the culprit as to what prompted an individual's seizure. Convulsions (twitching and shaking), intermittent cessation of breathing, loss of consciousness, etc. are all included, potentially, when someone has a seizure. An unsightly occurrence is the biting down on one's tongue during their seizure involuntarily. I've been on calls where the patient clenched their teeth down so hard on their tongue that I was afraid they were going to bite it off! When you start to see blood gushing from their tongue, you tend to think about these sorts of things.

Jeff and I were trying our hardest to find a residence located on a dirt road. Across from the strip of houses was a small canal that we had to maintain awareness of when turning our big ambulance around. We usually use a "backer" (someone who gets out and backs the ambulance driver up, usually a fireman, Jeff or myself) to avoid ditches, canals, buildings, signs and most importantly — people. One agency implemented an automatic termination policy if a supervisor spotted a unit backing up without a backer. They were so avid about enforcing this discipline because a civilian had actually died at the ambulance headquarters due to not using a backer. It was a real tragic death. Imagine dying by a huge truck slowly squashing your ribs, brains and guts like a bug!

Anyway, we identified our house and parked our unit just passed the driveway. This parking preference is put into play on most calls because when we wheel patients down the driveway, the ambulance is already positioned perfectly to load patients in the rear doors of the unit. Due to our call notes advising us that our patient was actively seizing, we made haste towards the entrance of the house. Someone from the occupancy had left the front door slightly open. Jeff began to advance passed the door's threshold when a wonderfully tattooed woman in a black wife beater appeared. She frantically yelled, "She won't stop shaking! She won't stop shaking! It started about 10 minutes ago! She hasn't stopped since then… only for a few seconds at a time!" Taking in what the woman said, Jeff and I briskly advanced passed her to see a smaller woman experiencing a full-body seizure on the ground. She had a multitude of tattoos as well. She had a very short haircut, almost like a boy haircut. "Has she ever had a seizure before?" I asked the woman who was in a panic. "Yes she's a regular for these things!" The woman replied with a large vein bulging from her temple. Jeff placed an oxygen cannula in the patient's nostrils. He then vigorously tossed our medication box to me so that I could prepare for an IV.

Glancing at her arms, I saw no veins — no veins at all. "Maybe a tourniquet, once applied, will raise them in to view" I thought. I applied the tourniquet tightly around her upper arm and waited briefly for veins to appear— still nothing. Undoing the tourniquet from her left upper arm, I quickly applied it tightly to her right upper arm. I waited briefly for a decent blood vessel to appear, but still none did. Just before I took my eyes away from searching her arm, a tiny vein came into view. This was the only vein available to work with. Taking out the proper needle size, I went for it. "No!" I thought in frustration. My attempt was unsuccessful! All the while our female patient was convulsing on the floor. She needed 5 mg of Valium, but I had not been able to establish the IV. I hate to say that we hurled our patient, but we picked her up from the floor and hurled her onto our stretcher. We had one last ditch effort to bank on — the rectal route.

Valium can be given through the rectum, so we prepared the dosage to be administered. "Help me turn her over onto her right side!" I yelled to Jeff. There we were — now in the rear of the ambulance fumbling around with medications, syringes and needles, struggling to get this young woman's trousers down to give her the Valium. Jeff spread her buttocks to give me a straight shot. In went the Valium up her rectum in one super push on the plunger of my syringe. We quickly pulled back up her pants and rolled her back onto her spine. The Valium kicked in a few moments later and she stopped seizing. Her skin was so pale that you would have thought she was a ghost! Bullets of sweat occupied almost the entire surface area of her skin. The shirt she wore turned two shades darker from all of the sweating; it went from the original light gray color to a dark metallic gray. Her hair looked as if she had just stepped out of the shower. This woman was completely exhausted. When you are violently jerking around for a long period of time, you lose a lot of energy. You can burn up a lot of blood glucose in your body as well. So we checked her blood sugar by way of pricking her index finger for a drop of blood to place in our glucometer (blood sugar measuring device). It turns out that it was very low. I drew up an ampule of glucagon to give her; this would raise her blood glucose level.

By the time she woke completely back up, we were pulling into the hospital. "Do you know where you're at miss?" I kindly asked her. She glared at me with a baffled face and slowly shook her head no. "What's the name of the city you live in?" I followed up. She maintained a puzzled look and gently raised her head on the head of the stretcher. She was what's called *postictal*. Patients who undergo seizures can get very confused and disoriented afterward. "Okay, inside we go… time to be evaluated by a doctor!" I said in a concluding manner. Another seizure had been stabilized, now it was a matter of getting blood work done to evaluate more sophisticated measures such as the possible imbalance of her cardiac enzymes.

Ye shall walk in all the ways which the Lord your God hath commanded you, that ye may live, and that it may be well with you, and that ye may prolong your days in the land which ye shall possess. **Deuteronomy 5:33**

#32

Butt Naked On The Bathroom Floor

Paramedic Pointer» The initial stages (infancy) and final stages (geriatric) of human life have something in common, which is decreased ability to regulate body temperatures. Both infants and senior citizens experience difficulty in regulating their temperatures. This is why the elderly enjoy warmer temperatures in their homes.

So you're going about your business on a regular day when it gets interrupted by some anonymous guy who has been reported to be sprawled out on the floor just outside the shower — butt naked. This is how emergency medical services works. It's simply the nature of the business. You can be having lunch, thinking of how good your meal is and immediately after, walk into an atrocious situation. You can be on the phone with your loved ones laughing it up and suddenly have to deal with a dying child. There's no saying, "I didn't sign up for this" or "This isn't fair." The fact of the matter is that you are there and you must perform sufficiently. Ever changing conditions is what makes this profession so exciting. Unlike a desk job, it's a lot harder to predict what's going to happen within a shift. You can guess all you want as a paramedic, but there's just no telling! What happened last shift will never happen again, at least not in the same way. There will be new faces involved, new houses, new injuries and different medical illnesses than the prior shift. Oh, the joys of being a paramedic! One must stay alert and aware because predictability is at a minimum in this line of work.

"Man down" is what was generated on the ambulance's dispatch screen. Immediately my mind began to jog, surveying the multitude of possibilities. Man down could mean anything between sleeping and dead. Further notes came in moments later, revealing that he was unconscious on the bathroom floor with no clothes on. Our response time was approximately four minutes. What we rolled up on was nothing short of a mansion. Guarding the double doors at the front were two lion statues exposing their sharp incisors with mouths wide open. Walking through those initial double doors revealed a spiral staircase going up to the occupant's second floor. "He's up here!" An older woman's voice rang out from above the winding stairwell. Jeff and I paced up the spiral stairs with our treatment bags in hand. Traveling upstairs always gave paramedic crews a decent workout because our bags are hefty!

Making it to that second floor provided a bit of relief to Jeff and I. The only light on the second floor must have been where our patient was. Out came an elderly woman with white hair that resembled smooth, white ribbon. She had crystal blue eyes that seemed as though they saw right through you. "My husband is in there," she said pointing towards the lighted bathroom while holding her silk robe with her other hand. "I was in the bedroom watching television when I heard a loud clunk!" she continued. Blood was everywhere. Not only did the bathroom floor have blood on it, but the side of the tub had blood smears too, as well as the wall. Blood was coming from the man's forehead. It seemed as if the man hit his head in the shower, touched the spot he hit on his head, freaked out from seeing blood and rushed out the shower, falling a second time. This gentleman lay restlessly with a fresh white towel halfway wrapped around his waist. He too had silky white hair with a thin white snow mustache to match it. His eyebrows were the same bright white color too. I began hooking the elderly gentleman up to our cardiac wires and the blood pressure cuff. Everything, unfortunately, was decreased. His heart rate was low. His blood pressure was low. His breathing was even decreased.

He intermittently gave out a brief grown as I speedily ran my short diagnostic tests. He was in a dangerous condition called symptomatic bradycardia, which in layman's terms means "low heart rate with other serious symptoms". Our drug of choice would be a medication called atropine. Atropine is a powerful drug; it's a real pleasure to watch take effect. Jeff managed the gentleman's bleeding with a sterile stack of gauze; I gained intravenous access in the patient's forearm. "How does his 12 lead (electrical picture of the heart) look?" Jeff asked. What he was concerned about, in all actuality, was not whether or not his heart was still pumping or not, but rather whether certain sophisticated activity was present that would hinder giving the atropine.

Every drug we give has its guidelines. Meeting our protocols criteria for giving atropine, I pushed it into my established IV. A fireman, who anxiously perused the bags for oxygen upon walking into our soirée, asked where we needed him. "If you would, go ahead and hang the normal saline 1000 mL bag so we can dump fluids into this gentleman," I said. Atropine began to prove its usefulness shortly after it was administered. Thankfully, it raised the gentleman's heart rate as it was manufactured to do. In addition, our fluids began to raise the white-haired patient's blood pressure. But what caused this abnormal decrease in his vital signs? What caused this man to fall? Did he grow faint or weak and just failed to hold himself up? Maybe he simply slipped — it is slippery inside a shower after all.

These are the kinds of questions paramedics must consider. Treating what is in front of you is nice and all, but learning the back story, or *history* of what has happened can reveal a whole host of valuable information. He ended up taking an excessive amount of cardiac inhibiting medication that inadvertently caused him to grow weak on top of plummeting his heart rate and blood pressure — that was the culprit. Jeff and I wrapped him up as decently as we could and performed a dead lift in getting him onto our cot. We managed to clean up most of the bleeding with bandages and cling wraps. Our elderly gentleman was also soaking wet, however. Him being wet wasn't of great concern beyond the risks it presented while lifting him— and that was already accomplished. Stabilizing him bought us time, but there was no way of measuring if this "stabilization" was temporary or permanently fixed. The white-haired gentleman needed to see an ER doctor for a full workup. The piece of equipment we plopped him down on was called a stair chair. You're not going to get an entire stretcher up the stairwell, certainly not a spiral stairwell. A stair chair contains tracks on the posterior of the chair so that you can lean it back and glide down a case of stairs. It also has wheels on it for moving the patient with ease.

There we were, going down in circles around and around again on the spiral staircase. With the white-haired gentleman strapped firmly into the chair, a fireman stabilizing the foot of the chair and myself on the backside, we advanced cautiously all the way down to the floor. A second fireman awaited us with the stretcher ready for the patient to be transferred on to from the stair chair. As soon as we made the transfer onto our cot, it was time to zoom. Baseline vitals were taken and critical interventions were already implemented. All there was left to do was close monitoring of an already stable patient en route to the ER. Off we went once our fellow fireman closed the back doors to our rig.

For not the hearers of the law are just before God, but the doers of the law shall be justified. **Romans 2:13**

#33

My Face Is Stuck!

Paramedic Pointer» *Baseline vital signs include: blood pressure, heart rate, respiratory rate and blood glucose (blood sugar).*

Ever not been able to move a particular part of your body? Sure, many of us know what it is to have a charlie horse and sit still until it subsides, but I'm talking about something a bit more alarming than a charlie horse. Imagine your *neck* locking up to the point that you cannot turn left or right — even if you force it with all your might! Imagine having a fixated gaze on an object that you cannot take your eyes off of, no matter how hard you tried! These are definitely out of the ordinary occurrences, but they do exist. If you are on antipsychotic meds (bless your heart if you are) this could become a reality for you. When people are prescribed to antipsychotic meds, a side effect known to happen occasionally is a phenomenon known as *dystonia*. Dystonia is marked by awkward facial contortions and muscle spasms.

A fellow by the name of Andre experienced this reaction late one night on his couch while watching television. As you may conclude, 911 was activated, which sent Jeff and I to his house like we were delivery boys. Though we were ordered, in a sense, we weren't delivering a pizza — not by a longshot. Andre was a 22-year-old African American male that sat gazing at the ceiling fan out of the corner of his eyes. His eyes were seemingly lodged into the upper left corners of his eye sockets as his head was tilted to the right at almost a

90° angle. It appeared as if his neck was broken. Another observer might be reminded of a zombie — Andre would certainly look possessed if you saw him walking down a dark corridor with minimal lighting. "He's been like this for about 20 minutes now", said a young black woman wearing a nightgown and a hair wrap. "Has this ever happened to him before?" I shot back quickly. "Not that I know of", replied the young woman. Attention turned to Andre as he desperately attempted to utter a barely discernible sentence. "My… face… is stuck…"He murmured. He clearly had somewhat control over his tongue and mouth. "What medications does Andre take, Miss? What kind of medical history does he have, if any?" I asked the young black woman who swayed side to side in a panicky motion. "Um… He has issues up here" she explained while tapping her index finger on her temple twice. "Got it" I answered back. I cut her off before she could finish her sentence because I could pick up on the vibe she was giving off — she didn't want to say something that sounded offensive such as "he's a little coo-coo".

Understanding now that he had a history of behavioral issues (a term medical professionals use to refer to psychiatric issues) I began weighing in the options that Andre was on antipsychotic drugs. Jeff and I both knew the symptoms Andre was experiencing were potentially stemming from the use of these kinds of medications. "Do you see any good veins, Jeff?" "Absolutely… this young man has got pipes for veins! I could stick him with an IV needle from across the room… like darts!" Jeff sprang into action as he knelt down to tear through our medical bags for a tourniquet and a needle. "I won't really need this but I'll use it anyway for good measure," Jeff said as he dangled the blue tourniquet in front of his face like a giant string of spaghetti. Andre's veins were so prominent that they already did what a tourniquet is meant to elicit— bulge. "Done…that was incredibly easy," Jeff boasted.

"Draw up 50 mg of Benadryl, if you would, Jeff," I directed. Benadryl was the answer for dystonic reactions such as this. The automatic blood pressure cuff was counting down on the opposite arm of the IV line. We waited for a brief period for the blood pressure cuff to finish so that we could see where his blood pressure rested. It came back normal. A quick touch of Andre's wrist elicited a normal pulse range to Jeff, who did the honors of checking his heart rate. I made sure Andre was not allergic to Benadryl and gave the go ahead to Jeff to push the medication. "I can't move my face," mumbled Andre for a second time, relaying his dilemma to us. "We're doing everything we can to help that as we speak, Andre," I assured him. His face was still stuck in an awkward contortion and you could see the terror in his eyes. Everything from his neck up was frozen. His eyes, at the moment, were still immovable from the upper left corners of his eye sockets. He was probably fearful that he would be stuck this way forever.

That's downright cruelty on top of cruelty if this was to result in permanence. The torturing bondage would cause one to go mad. For Andre, it would cause him to go even *more* mad since he was already on antipsychotic meds. "The 50 mg of Benadryl is in!" Jeff announced. No instant results came about. We allowed a few moments to pass. Still no relief from the dystonic reaction. Jeff and I shot each other an uneasy look and began preparing to place Andre on our stretcher. "My neck is stiff… I can't move my head at all" our patient managed to say through clenched teeth. Had you been on the scene, you would have witnessed the same look of despair that paralyzed Jeff and I. It brings to mind a scene from a horror movie called the *Wish Master* where a woman was turned into a mannequin. All she could move was her eyeballs. Andre endured the discomfort with as much patience as he could, but one could tell that his patience, and not to mention, sanity, was wearing thin.

Tension grew as time moved forward. A single stream of lacrimation traveled down Andre's left cheek. Would he be like this forever? Certainly the likelihood of this had to be extremely low, but entertaining the thought alone would make one cringe. Further, things have a way of creating a sense of impending doom when you're the one in the hot seat— or in this case— the seat of the stretcher.

Arriving at the hospital marked a breakthrough. Driving from the patient's house to the hospital took about five minutes — a timeframe that can feel like a lifetime under emergency conditions. Andre first regained control of his eye movements. My heart dropped. "Thank goodness," I thought to myself. Next, his head dropped straight down, his chin sinking into his chest. It appeared as if some sort of hex had been lifted and Andre was depleted of being controlled all in an instant. He slowly lifted his head, resting it on the head of the stretcher in contentment. He blinked a couple of times and looked up, down and all around in circles, making sure that he was completely back to his normal self again. He was back alright. The medication proved to be successful in providing a solution! With a hand placed on Andre's shoulder, I said, "Welcome back, it's good to see you back in control over your own body." He smiled and emitted a sigh of relief as the stretcher wheels rolled towards the automatic sliding ER doors.

Verily, verily, I say unto you, he that hears my word, and believeth on him that sent me, hath everlasting life, and shall not come into condemnation; but is passed from death unto life. **John 5:24**

#34

Bear Down!

Paramedic Pointer» *More so a concern in elderly patients, one can actually pass out from bearing down (straining to move bowels) for too long on the toilet. The medical term is called vagal maneuvers. We instruct patients with very high heart rates to attempt vagal maneuvers because it can effectively decrease their heart rates.*

Before going into a restaurant by the name of *Zeko's*, the skies were immaculately clear. It was dinner time, a florescent sunset graced the city with its charming glamour. We had just zipped over to a Mexican restaurant (trailer on wheels) that my partner visited on a regular basis. I was after an entrée of delectable chicken wings and potato fries. A rule in EMS is to eat your fries first because you may get a call, and we all know fries are ruined after they cool down. It's just the universal truth that reheated fries are a no no. The same rule goes for hash browns in the morning time. Paramedics are always on the bubble for another call. It could happen at any moment, and the good citizens of the world could care less if you're having dinner or whatever else you may be doing.

Thankfully we managed to complete both of our meals. There was no rushing to scarf down the last few bites for either of us (Jeff and I). What's worse than having to rush your food down is when you mistakenly pay for the entrée first, receive a call from dispatch, and then have to bolt with *no* food. You end up simply donating cash to some random restaurant. However, there is another position a paramedic ends up in at some point or another — hopefully not too frequently. It was the position I happen to be in on this beautiful evening. Following a fantastic meal with my partner, my tank was full and I needed to offload. I'm not only referring to draining the main vein, but also going number two. Like women, this requires us to sit down. If you still haven't decoded my casual clues then I'll say it plainly — I was *pooping* when an emergency call came in. I had just started, so inevitably, I needed to shut down the chocolate factory before I was ready. And remember the entrancing sunset the Florida skies had granted us? Yeah, well, somehow in a matter of 40 minutes, that tranquil sunset had morphed into a windy rainstorm! So not only would I be getting drenched on the way to the ambulance, but I would have to manage a condition called "mudd butt" on the scene of this current call.

Hopping into a flickering ambulance (Jeff was already in the driver seat with the emergency lights on), I keyed up the mic to verbalize "Going en route" to our call. Traffic was backed up as we advanced towards the location. This wasn't even our zone, to my surprise — our zone never allowed us to cover for another unit's zone because we were the busiest call zone in the entire county of Manatee. Inching passed long, crowded lines of cars that could barely move, brought us to an apartment complex. Blue and red lights lit up the now dark gray skies. Each raindrop next to the cop cars on scene reflected the blue and red, making for a brilliant show of watercolors. In the midst of about four police officers stood a middle-aged caucasian woman. She was pale white with short choppy hair. She gave no real facial expression, just sort of a bland stare off into the distance as if she had no care in the world. Policemen were already on the scene because there was suspicion of illegal drug use. "What is your name?" I said, looking directly at our soon-to-be patient.

"Who me?" The woman said. My question caused her to snap out of her daydreaming. Being able to daydream in the rain probably isn't impossible, but there sure is an index of suspicion when you're doing it on a rainy evening among four officers and two paramedics. "My name is Mary," she said. "Come on and step inside my unit so we can evaluate you inside. My name is Lorenzo and this is my partner Jeff, we'll be your paramedics for the day. Now tell me, what exactly is going on today?" "I'm experiencing withdrawal from drugs. I've used heroin for many many years and my body doesn't know how to respond now that I've given it up." Here's something that you don't see very often. Someone who has decided that enough is enough in regards to their addiction. "Congratulations, Mary, for taking a giant leap in deciding to better yourself," I commended her. "What kind of symptoms are you having today?" "I've thrown up about three times today, my head hurts, and my heart is racing uncontrollably! I can feel a fluttering sensation... I'm so scared!" As I interviewed Mary, Jeff applied our diagnostic tools to her body. He applied a blood pressure cuff, a pulse oximeter (finger probe to monitor pulse) and cardiac wires to monitor the activity in her heart. Her heart was racing all right! Normal heart rates span from 60 bpm to 100 bpm— Mary's heart rate was 168! Jeff shot me a worried look from behind the head of the stretcher. He sat in the captain's chair, which lied just beyond Mary's head. She was facing me, so she was blissfully unaware of the concerned look that came over Jeff's face upon seeing her heart rate on the monitor.

"Okay, we're going to move quickly in doing a few things, Mary, because you're heart rate is very fast," I informed the pale woman as she sat shivering on my stretcher. We turned off the AC and gave Mary a blanket to warm her up. "I want you to bear down and hold it for a few seconds," I instructed her. "What do you mean? Strain as if I'm trying to have a bowel movement?" "Exactly," I replied. The irony of what I was doing in the bathroom of that Zeko's restaurant came to mind as I coached Mary through a procedure medically known as vagal maneuvers. Vagal maneuvers are sometimes effective in lowering an individual's heart rate by bearing down, mimicking an attempt to move bowels. "Her heart rate has decreased to a rate of 158!" Blurted Jeff. This was a positive sign. The negative aspect of it, however, was that it was still outside of normal ranges — by far.

"Breakout the adenosine!" I directed Jeff while pointing to the medication cabinet. Being one of my favorite drugs, adenosine has a very interesting mechanism of action. It slows conduction through the AV node in your heart. In other words, the end-all result of this drug is just like hitting the reset button on a PlayStation or an Xbox. It literally will *reset* your heart, so to speak, and recalibrate the pumping of your cardiac muscle. Oh, and one more ridiculously cool thing about this drug you should know: when adenosine resets one's heart, the patient experiences 2-3 seconds of being *flat line* on the cardiac monitor. So, in a way, people who receive this drug end up being dead for about two seconds!

While Jeff prepared the adenosine, I coached Mary once more at a second attempt to lower her heart rate with vagal maneuvers. Again, her heart rate lowered, but not enough. "Everything's ready to go!" Jeff notified me. Being handed the loaded syringe, I quickly began twisting it on to the established IV in her left forearm—I had just completed gaining IV access during the second coaching session of vagal maneuvers. Slamming the medication in, Jeff and I gathered to observe the monitor for that *flat line* phenomenon. About five seconds passed and the monitor revealed what we expected to see. No cardiac waveform on the monitor screen, just a long motionless line spanning from one side to the next, all the way across. (This is an occurrence we typically don't show patients because it's downright creepy if you're the one it's happening to!). Moments later, Mary's heart returned to a strong 70 beats per minute (normalcy).

Now Mary felt nauseous. "I think I'm going to throw up you guys, do you have a basin?" "We sure do… here you are," I said, handing Mary a convenience bag (vomit bag). She barked up a slew of orangish-red vomit two seconds after being handed the convenience bag. "I guess that calls for a vial of Zofran," concluded Jeff. "We're going to give you something to help your nausea and then we'll get going." Glancing at our monitor revealed Mary's heart maintaining steadily at 70 beats per minute. Mary's heart was back to normal. After giving her Zofran, her nausea would be in check as well. Jeff took off his purple medical gloves and threw them in the trash can; he was getting ready to jump up front to drive. "I'll take the road nice and smooth, Mary, I promise. Another thing I promise is that you're in good hands, that ain't no doubt! I'll see you both at the ER," Jeff said before exiting the patient compartment. It gave us both relief that we would be transporting a now stable patient.

And the work of righteousness shall be peace; and the effect of righteousness quietness and assurance forever. **Isaiah 32:17**

#35

Sudden Death

Paramedic Pointer» *Criteria for pronouncing a patient "dead" includes: rigor mortis (stiffness), no breathing/pulse, lividity (blood pooling at the bottom of the body), cold to the touch and a flat line waveform on the cardiac monitor. Being cold and stiff signifies an extended time period of being dead, prompting paramedics to not begin resuscitative efforts.*

Death visits each and every one of us. No man (or woman) knows the year, month, day, hour, minute or moment he or she will take their last breath. I've walked into nursing home rooms where patients have literally gasped for their last breath as I walked through the door. I've seen lives of spouses taken right before their significant others' eyes. If I didn't value a person's life, I wouldn't have signed up for this line of work, so I do not wish to discount the value of anyone's life with my next statement. What I would like to extend to you is that there is something greater than your existence here on earth. What I'm talking about, that is greater than a breath, greater than a heartbeat, is the importance of your soul.

As a Christian, I believe that the life lived here on earth is only an *audition* for eternity. Whenever I come across a patient who passes away inevitably before my eyes, my mind ponders whether that particular individual came to know Christ or not. Everything done under the sun is granted by God. We are all privileged to walk this earth and enjoy the laughter, anger and tears it comes with. As one who cares for you, please make sure your heart is in the right place to the best of your ability and remember to thank God for all that you have, for no one knows when their last heartbeat is going to happen. Deaths are not tragic. True tragedy is a soul not saved by Jesus Christ before one's time on earth lapses.

Cardiac arrests are the precise calls where paramedics can potentially make the biggest turnaround. For those of you not familiar with the term, I'll define it in a short and sweet fashion. There are two short phrases you'll need to remember when recalling the definition of cardiac arrest and they are: 1) *no breathing* and 2) *no pulse*. Now you know why I say they are the most prominent emergency calls paramedics can make the biggest turnaround on! We paramedics, using electricity (defibrillation), drugs and airway management can potentially transform a dead patient into a live patient. It's not a satisfaction guarantee; many factors must align. Factors such as: timing, teamwork, skill and yes, a bit of luck at times.

Jeff and I received a call for a "man slumped over in the driver seat of his Buick." Dispatch notified us that his wife was the one who called. She was sitting in the passenger seat with their two adult children occupying the two back seats. When we arrived, the older gentleman was indeed leaning forward against his steering wheel. His Buick was parked perfectly in the driveway, so I assume they had just got in the car to leave or just got home getting ready to get out of the car. All in all, it could've been worse for everyone in the vehicle had dad lost consciousness while the car was moving in traffic!

We approached the silver Buick briskly; the wife conveyed a terrified look, progressing to tear shed, and the adult children appeared baffled at everything that was going on. Jeff opened the driver door and extended his index and middle fingers toward the man's neck to feel a pulse. "I've got no pulse!" urged Jeff. "Get prepared for a *CODE*!" Jeff demanded. A fire truck responded to this call as well — firemen responded to calls that could possibly demand extra help such as this one. On scene were a total of three firemen, myself and Jeff. Two of the three firemen snatched our patient out of the driver seat and laid him flat on the driveway pavement. One fireman locked his elbows and began to initiate CPR on the coded patient (code means cardiac arrest). Gurgles were heard shortly after CPR started, it proved to be blood pooling in the patient's mouth. "I need suction!" I shouted in a hurry. A fireman scurried to the head of the patient, precisely where I was positioned on both knees. 10 seconds of aggressive suctioning turned out to be sufficient enough to clear the patient's airway— I needed it to be free of obstruction in order to successfully intubate him. Intubation is an advanced airway intervention that involves placing a breathing tube down a person's windpipe. Intubation allows care providers to breathe for a patient by squeezing a connected oxygen bag.

"Administer the epinephrine!" I directed Jeff, who had started an IV in the patient's left arm where the arm bends at, opposite of the elbow. "First round of epi has been given!" confirmed Jeff. So now we had vigorous CPR in motion, an established IV for drugs and what would soon be an airway that was completely under control. Opening up the patient's mouth to attempt an intubation revealed an *increasing* amount of blood filling up slowly. "I need to suction his mouth one more time and then I'll go for it!" I said in realizing the gradual blood increase within the patient's throat. Another seven seconds of aggressive suctioning took place by my hand. Directly after I put the suction unit down, I put the tube into the patient's mouth and secured it. "It's time for a round of amiodarone!" I announced. Right there in the neighborhood driveway, five medical personnel (us) worked diligently to preserve a man's life. Glancing upward at the wife and kids, his wife's eyes were filled with tears. She covered her opened mouth with both of her hands. The male child embraced his sister in the midst of the calamity.

"Do we have a pulse?" I loudly questioned. Jeff concentrated, blocking out the surrounding commotion as he felt the patient's neck and wrist simultaneously. "No... No pulse yet!" He said with reluctance. "After the next pulse check, I'll need someone to rotate with me on CPR," said a fireman who worked up a decent sweat from manually pumping on our patient's chest. "Everyone clear?!" I yelled. "All clear!" Everyone replied. "Charging... Charging...aaannnnddd... shock delivered!" I announced after sending electricity through the patient. Everyone immediately jumped back on CPR, drug administration and general care of the breathless patient. "Were almost out of epinephrine," Jeff advised. "Here's the last vile, I'm pushing it in now!" We carried on with *working* the patient to see if we could revive him. Our fight was fought strategically and skillfully, but it was time to call it quits. There was no chance of bringing this gentleman back, his fate was sealed shut.

"NOOOOO!!!" Cried the wife. "CARL!!!" She continued. The on scene crew allowed her to mourn her loss. Compassionately addressing the loss, I said to the lady, "I'm truly sorry. We did everything we could." My crew gathered all of the trash from the mess we made. Two of the firemen draped white sheets over the male patient's corpse to retain decency. There was nothing left to be said or done about this unfortunate event. The coroner would be by in a matter of time.

There shall no evil befall thee, neither shall any plague come nigh thy dwelling. For he shall give his angels charge over thee, to keep thee in all thy ways. **Psalm 91:10 – 11**

#36

Metabolic Madness

Paramedic Pointer» *High blood sugar, when high enough, can be just as destructive as low blood sugar.*

Zone 16, today, had been a wonderful whirlwind of ongoing emergencies. One after another the emergency calls fell upon us like raindrops. Zone 16 provided plenty to stay busy with for the full duration of my 24 hours on duty. Throughout the day we ran our butts off. Overnight, well, you were lucky if you snuck four hours of sleep in— total. If you've ever watched a NASCAR race then you can compare the repetitiveness of a NASCAR race to this day. Just as you may get dizzy from watching all the cars go round and round in circles, our call volume was so high that it made my head spin.

"I'm going to try and get something to eat before we get another call," Jeff said to me as we pulled into a local diner. "What do you plan on getting?" I questioned. "I'm in the mood for a good ol' American cheeseburger and fries," Jeff exclaimed. Just as Jeff's hand grabbed the diner's entrance door handle, we were notified of a call. I saw Jeff jerk his head forward in disappointment — and rightfully so. We must of been on our ninth call of the day, neither of us had the chance to eat since just before call number one. I had small snacks from the hospital here and there when I could. Each hospital provides a complementary EMS room out of appreciation for public safety personnel. These rooms are typically stocked with snack food and beverages. What perplexed me about these rooms was that they often only kept sodas in their inventories. As someone who primarily drinks water and Gatorade, it was a nightmare for me. Jeff's stomach had to be so empty that it was touching his back. Peanuts, cheez-its and small premade PB&J's held my hunger in check. Jeff whipped the ambulance driver door open and pulled himself up into the driver seat. Adjusting his steering wheel, he asked, "What's on the menu?" referring to the type of emergency we were to respond to. "We'll be heading to a 66-year-old female, unconscious, who is experiencing diabetic problems," I answered Jeff.

Placing the Ambo (Ambulance) in gear, Jeff nodded at my statement with his neon sunglasses on and mashed the gas pedal. Bending a few corners and scaling a couple roundabouts, Jeff grew a bit flustered. "My God, Lorenzo, why won't these idiots move out of the way? Do they not hear the sirens? Do they not hear my loud air horn when it's clearly audible? Do they not see with their own eyes this humongous vehicle we're in that's lighting up??" he said in a frantic, irritated voice. Jeff proceeded to stomp on the loud air horn and hold it for three seconds at a time in the midst of frustration. "Some people just don't hear apparently!" Jeff muttered. Do not be misled, Jeff is a great guy, it's just that his hunger was getting the best of him. Patience tends to run thin when you're both tired *and* hungry.

Minutes later, we came up to a small trailer where firemen were entering as we slowed to a stop. Gathering our supplies, I handed Jeff a pair of gloves, hoping that he had calmed down a bit. A fireman came right back out to greet us, saying, "I'm going to tell you right now, you guys won't be able to fit the stretcher in here partner! They are hoarders, there's only enough room for bodies to fit through the pathways, and even with just our bodies it's a tight fit in there!" The fireman gave me a slight look of distress as he shook his head slowly with his hands on his hips. "I think our best bet is gonna be to bring the patient out on a bed sheet, she's just a little old lady. We checked her blood sugar and it was severely low!" Jeff and I, still standing just outside the front door, agreed with his suggested method of bringing the old woman out, who was unconscious. He rushed back inside to retrieve the little old woman with the other two firemen. You would've thought our female patient was dead, as pale as she was. They carried her out on a white sheet, holding the ends such that it looked as if she was merely sleeping peacefully in a hammock. "Get her inside the ambulance fast", I encouraged everyone on scene, buckling her into our cot simultaneously.

Locking her into place so that the stretcher would not slide around in the back of the Ambo, I made my way to the IV start kit, ripping open the packaging. Her blood sugar was dangerously low, top priority rested on getting an intravenous line established so that a medication could be given. In emergencies involving low blood sugar, we administer a drug named *dextrose*. It is essentially liquid sugar, prepared to be safely given in one's bloodstream. "Is your IV good?" Jeff asked. "Absolutely — one and done" I boasted. I was referring to the number of attempts because it's not always a guarantee that you will get the IV the first time with all patients. As much as we paramedics would like for this to be the case, certain patients can have poor veins. "The full ampule of dextrose has been pushed," I told Jeff. "Did you give half the ampule or the entire 25 g?" "25 g" I assured Jeff. We sat quietly no longer than two minutes until our patient regained consciousness before our eyes.

She returned to being alert with accelerated breathing. She looked around in awe, "Where am I? How long was I out?" She questioned. "Your husband says you lost consciousness about 10 minutes before we arrived," I answered. "Have you had anything to eat today?" "No," the old woman replied. "I was working out in my yard, planting seeds in my garden since this morning. When I came back inside, I do vaguely remember feeling ill." "No wonder your body's sugar was low, you haven't eaten anything all day!" I chuckled lightheartedly. "I don't want to go to the hospital, I'm fine," the little old woman looked up and proclaimed. "This dextrose isn't going to uphold your sugar for long, Miss. It will last for about 30 – 45 minutes, but that's about it. If you're going to sign a refusal, you'll need to eat something… some complex carbs like a glass of milk and PB&J." "Okay, my husband can make some for me in a jippy if you don't mind."

"Absolutely," I replied. Indeed her hubby prepared a gourmet peanut butter and jelly sandwich that our patient devoured. We allowed her to stay home since the sandwich would retain a normal blood glucose level. "All we need now is a signature from you, Miss," I exclaimed. The small elderly woman signed our computer screen and sat back down at her kitchen table. "Call us back if you need us, by all means, okay?" I advised. "You guys are great… I sure will".

Then shalt thou call, and the Lord shall answer; thou shalt cry, and he shall say, here I am. **Isaiah 58:9**

#37

Three Strikes and You're Out —But It Only Takes One Stroke

Paramedic Pointer» *A strong precursor to a stroke is the patient claiming to have "The worst headache of his or her life." This is due to the extremely high blood pressures that accompany strokes.*

Altered mental status can be a result of anything. You could have an altered mental status because you were hit over the head with a baseball bat. You can have altered mental status because you're drunk. So many different possibilities arise when it comes to diagnosing an individual's altered mental status. The culprit is found only in investigation — medical investigation that is. A paramedic must find out what the events leading up to the emergency was, medications taken by the patient and general medical history of that particular patient. When we paced through the front door of an older African-American male's house, we saw a patient who looked severely confused.

In fact, his mouth was wide open with a stream of drool falling from his chin. He stared at the wall with this fixated gaze that made you feel he was in some sort of hypnotic trance. The television was on but he wasn't staring at the television. His blank stare gave off no indication that he was aware of his surroundings. "I'm so glad you all are here! This is my husband, Ted. I noticed that he didn't respond to me when I called him from the kitchen!" Ted's wife cried. "How long ago did you call for him?" "About five minutes ago. I came out here to the living room and found him just sitting here like he is now. I tried to get his attention several times with no response! That's when I got scared and called you guys. This is not like him at all. Not ever. He's usually playful 24 hours, seven days a week. He's always the first one to crack a joke too." Following the acknowledgment of what the wife had explained, I turned to Ted and attempted to shake him gently while saying, "Hey Ted, can you hear me Sir?" No response. "Place the equipment on him and obtain a set of vitals," I directed Jeff. His wife scurried to the kitchen to gather Ted's prescribed medications. She returned before the automatic blood pressure cuff finished acquiring a blood pressure. "Here they are, there are only a few medications that he's on. One of them, I know, is for his high blood pressure. He's pretty healthy outside of that."

"His blood pressure is extremely elevated," Jeff informed me. "It seems he might be experiencing a stroke based off of his presentation," Jeff explained. "I'm going to perform a few tests quickly to see what's going on." I confiscated Ted's medications and rushed over to perform an IV. Ted was in another world, so to speak. He was anywhere but here on earth, that's for certain. "He has failed the stroke test! Let's get him packaged up (properly seat belted on our stretcher) and run him to the hospital now!" Jeff said hurriedly. With a blood pressure through the roof, altered mental status and right-sided weakness, it became apparent that Ted was undergoing a stroke.

"This is medic 16, we're paging you to activate a stroke alert at the hospital," I said, keying up my radio mic that rested on my hip. "Stroke alert recorded at 1800 hours," replied the dispatcher. By the time I was finished notifying our local hospital of a stroke patient soon to be *their* patient, Ted vomited all over my partner Jeff — it was projectile vomit! The way it shot out of Ted's mouth was like how a water hose bursts out upon someone squeezing the handle. Jeff had no time to dodge the scattergun of vomit. "This is just great!" Jeff said as he helped me move Ted onto our cot. Our three medical bags still sat on the ground in the living room. I threw the two bags over my left and right shoulder. Jeff snatched the remaining medical bag off of the floor as we spun the stretcher around to exit the residence feet first.

Ted's small house dog picked the perfect time to begin barking viciously and biting around my ankles. Ted's wife saw what the small dog was doing (probably out of protection for Ted) and scooped him up in a hurry. "Get over here Roxie! They're not going to hurt daddy, they want to help him!" she sweet talked the tiny dog, beginning to pet it's fur. With her intervention, the dog simmered down and accepted us taking its owner, whom apparently the dog cared deeply for. "We'll be going to the nearest hospital Miss, thanks for all your help." "I'll be following right behind you in a moment; I'll be seeing you there!" Ted's wife yelled in a concerned tone. Jeff and I rushed Ted out to our rig, cutting directly through the front lawn. From the front door to our stretcher being completely locked into place inside our rig couldn't have taken any longer than 15 seconds.

"Let's get rolling!" I hollered at Jeff, who then raced to the driver seat for takeoff. Ted and I bounced up and down occasionally as we raced across raised potholes in the road. Ted vomited once more en route to the hospital, this time only minimally — no projectile barf the second time. I kept saying under my breath, "Hang in there Ted, hang in there…" Hoping that we could just get him inside the ER for an MRI. Every other moment, it seemed, I found myself reevaluating his airway, breathing and circulation. His overall condition did not change en route, the problem was that his condition, in it of itself was terrible. After all, strokes are nothing minute. Many *die* from strokes. On the other hand, many survive strokes but then there's the group that are pretty much just alive with no real awareness of their surroundings — senile, as they call it.

In conclusion, Ted's ER assessment revealed that he had a hemorrhagic stroke. In simpler terms, Ted had a bleed going on in his brain. No, I'm not sure what his final state would be, if he indeed survived that is. What I can tell you is that not all misfortunes get mended with a happy ending. That's the ugly truth of emergency medical services. Ted's wife was present at the ER as she promised — giving all her support that she could to her beloved husband.

*For thus saith the Lord unto the house of Israel, seek ye me, and ye shall live. **Amos 5:4***

#38

Brain Matter

Paramedic Pointer» *As corny as it may sound, always put safety first via seat belts, helmets and other protective garments needed for travel. The truth is: sometimes even these aren't enough. Defensive driving, as well, is a must.*

Somehow, you're driving into the wind feeling the breeze grace your skin and you lose control — out of nowhere a life-changing event occurs. It involves trauma — nasty trauma. Near-decapitation trauma. Who would have thought? People make mistakes while on the road, right? That's expected. Heck, people even lose control themselves, becoming their own worst nightmare. There are so many paths that lead to the same destruction. I guess the saying "There's more than one way to skin a cat" has truth to it.

Automobile accidents are obscenely frequent in the vast world we live in. I was told by a paramedic agency once that before we die, we will all have been in at least one vehicle wreck. The instructor of the class I heard that statistic from was a very short, stocky woman. Her name was Miss Debbie— she was a seasoned EMS professional. "If you've ever been in a vehicle collision, raise your hand," she told the class. I happened to be sitting high up in the stadium style auditorium, where I could see everyone in the room. After everyone heard her request, they all raised their hand — everyone but me. Miss Debbie said, "That's all of you. Everyone can expect to be in at least one vehicle collision/accident within their lifetime." I smiled and raised my hand. "Yes, Mr. Hogans?" Miss Debbie said with a raised brow behind her reading glasses. "Not me, I've never been in an automobile accident thus far." She gave a halfhearted grin and replied, "It's only a matter of time Mr. hogans… It's only a matter of time." Her words, spoken confidently, still replay in my head when I think about it. And they replay in slow motion oddly enough. I can hear them now — "It's only a matter of time… It's only a matter of time." Interestingly enough, I can say that Miss Debbie was right. My time, as she stated, has already passed. It happened just a few weeks following that public safety lecture when a crazy driver sideswiped me during an emergency response in the ambulance. How do you hit a lighted cube on wheels that makes an abundance of irritating noise? I couldn't believe it. It happened at a busy intersection I was making a left turn at. Jeff and I were en route to an auto accident, ironically, and *became* an auto accident. We ended up having to go *out of service* for hours, not to mention, another ambulance was forced to take our call. It was a mess.

Per company policy, Jeff and I had to be tested for alcohol/substance intoxication, even though we were the ones who were sideswiped! But this isn't a story about my seemingly prophetic vehicle accident. This story is about another vehicle accident involving a cyclist, which didn't end well, by the way. These particular cyclist accidents are the reasons why people have taken it upon themselves to create rear windshield placards that say, "Watch for motor-cycles." Another popular rear windshield placard you may have seen around town is the yellow placard that reads, "Baby on board." You know what I'm referring to, and if you don't, you may want to consider getting out more into the real world.

The bloody accident occurred smack dab in the middle of a causeway that connected main lands to the beach coast. Instead of your typical metal guard rails seen on the interstate, these guardrails were made of concrete. As soon as we arrived on scene of the call, we observed the remains of what use to be a motorcycle. This style motorcycle is often referred to as a "crotch rocket". It's the sporty kind younger guys and gals ride, unlike the Harley-Davidson cruiser older men in biker gangs enjoy. The crotch rocket was torn to shreds!

So was the patient's helmet, which was 75% missing from the patient's head. Helmet remains were scattered all over, along with the long trail of motorcycle remnants starting from the beginning of the causeway. My partner raced over to check a pulse on the motorcycle driver, who appeared to already be DOA (dead on arrival). "He's dead," Jeff acknowledged aloud. "Unsurvivable trauma," he added. Instead of continuing towards Jeff's direction, I turned in the opposite direction to head towards a Native American family standing next to an SUV. I casually observed the father of that family consoling his wife (holding her tightly against his chest) and two small children.

Opening my mouth to begin to speak, my foot got stuck. I looked down and picked my foot up, feeling a gum-like mass sticking to the bottom my shoe. Studying it closely, I realized that this was nowhere close to gum — not by a longshot. Peering more closely as I leaned down further, I made out that this sticky mass was brain matter. Glancing around my surroundings, I realized there was more of it strewn about. I knelt down after taking a few more steps forward, picking up another piece of brains with a gloved hand. It was sticky— unusually sticky. Brain matter has to be the absolute stickiest substance I've ever felt. Whenever you see one in a laboratory, it's either dried out or lubed up nicely. Not this one. Fresh out of the skull of a real human, brain matter is stickier than you would believe. I almost had to take my entire glove off to rid my hand of the brain matter that was stuck to it.

Our now deceased patient wore a helmet, so he must've been traveling at a pretty high speed to shatter a safety rated motorcycle helmet upon collision with the guard rail. As I walked closer to the guard rail, more brain matter became visible. The cyclist's brains were literally on each post I passed, signifying that he likely hit his head multiple times along the safety railing. Blood and brains were smeared everywhere I glanced. "How brutal of a bashing this fellow took to his head," I thought to myself. Finally I came to the Native American family who were frightened senselessly.

Everyone was uninjured and surprisingly not involved with the cyclist. "He swerved around my SUV at the speed of light and lost control," the trembling father said through his nervous lips. "What's happening with him? Is he alive?" asked the Native American father. "No," Jeff interjected, walking up to us. He incurred unsurvivable trauma, Sir," Jeff answered reluctantly. "His skull was shattered," Jeff whispered to me under his breath. "I'm glad you all are uninjured and symptom-free. Sign here please," I motioned the father of the family to sign my laptop. "Be safe Sir, have a safe rest of the night," I advised. The Native American family, still in shock, slowly got back into their SUV. "Can't save them all," Jeff muttered. "I know it, it's a real shame," I replied. "The old Grim Reaper got our patient this time around," Jeff joked lightheartedly. "You're right about that Jeff," I said shaking my head. "If only we could get the Grim Reaper… now *that* would be something."

But without faith it is impossible to please him: for he that cometh to God must believe that he is, and that he is a rewarder of them that diligently seek him. **Hebrews 11:6**

#39

The Loss Of a Life And The Loss Of a Wife

Paramedic Pointer» *Hold your loved ones a little bit tighter the next time you see them. Take advantage of each opportunity to show that you care; no man/woman knows the hour of which they will pass away.*

The pinnacle of awkwardness, discomfort, strange vibes and empathy was achieved on scene of a devastating call that resulted in one of two lives lost. A husband and wife tumbled down a busy road in a turbo golf cart. Like a normal golf cart, the vehicle had no doors or windows. All other attributes of a regular golf cart were comparable except for the gigantic tires this one had, coupled with the supercharged turbo speeds this particular golf cart seemed to have. As with most emergency calls, I was not there to witness the way things unfolded in real time. What I saw, as in most cases, was the *end result*. In this case, the end result was a slightly injured man and a female fatality.

Our ambulance tires stopped about 10 yards from an anonymous body lying in the middle of the busy street. Through the windshield of the ambulance I could see a puddle of dark red blood, slowly increasing in diameter, under the female patient's head. Her head rested lifelessly in that small pond of blood with no hint of any movement. "Let's grab everything including a backboard and our suction unit, it looks like we're going to be working a cardiac arrest," I said. While quickly collecting all of the necessary equipment, a fire truck rolled up, accompanied by dangerously loud noise. Its loud sirens abruptly shut off at the same time the long fire truck came to a complete halt.

Three firemen jumped out in bunker pants and red overalls looking for work to do. They walked in unison with my partner Jeff and I. A few short comments were made between the bunch of us but as we inched closer and closer to the downed female patient, silence grew. We knew the seriousness of our patient's state — she was obviously unconscious from a traumatic injury, but she may have already been dead. One of the firemen knelt down and assessed a pulse at the woman's neck, just below her left jaw. "I've got no pulse guys," the fireman advised, dropping his head down as if he had been defeated. "What do her pupils look like?" I asked intuitively. "They are big and wide… completely dilated," he answered. The same fireman reached around to feel the posterior portion of her head. "It feels like mush, my hand is just sinking into her head" the fireman relayed as he examined the patient. "Do you feel the skull? Is it cracked?" I questioned. "Yep, she cracked her head wide open when she hit the pavement, it must've been a really hard blow," he added.

"Go ahead and hook her up to our monitor so we can electronically document her cardiac rhythm," I urged. In placing her on our cardiac monitor, no activity was found, only a flat line spanning from the left side of the screen to the right. We captured the waveform on the monitor screen for a few seconds for documentation purposes. In order to maintain decency, we placed a white sheet over the female patient's body as she lay dead on the busy street. Both the firemen and my ambulance were parked strategically to block traffic. One lane was intentionally left open so that traffic could still get through, however.

Running from the sidewalk, a man sprinted with all of his might to the draped female. He uncovered the head portion of the sheet and began to experience a total meltdown. "Who are you sir? What are you doing?" An on-scene policeman asked aggressively. "NOOOOOO!!!!! WHY GOD?!?! OH NOOOOOOO!!!!" "Sir, are you the husband of this woman?" "EEYYYYEESSSS!!!! OH NO GOD…GOD…

NOOOO!!! NOT MY WIFE! I'M SOO SORRRYYY!!! I'M SO SORRYY HONEY!!!" The husband of the now dead patient slammed his fist on the concrete while kneeling on both knees. He pounded the pavement so hard that I thought he could have started an earthquake. He pounded and pounded in an emotionally charged fit of rage until his knuckles started to bleed. Meanwhile, the same officer who asked the man who he was, walked up to Jeff and I and said, "I smell a real strong odor coming from that guy, he reeks of alcohol!" My eyes widened when I heard him make this statement.

"You got to be kidding me," I thought. Here's a guy who accidentally killed his wife and did so while under the influence, potentially. "You have to test his blood/alcohol level now for sure. I'll need a blood draw from you if you don't mind," the officer turned to me and said. "No problem officer, you bet," I replied. Thankfully, the policeman allowed the devastated husband a few minutes of solitude to mourn his loss. The policeman walked over to the kneeling husband and placed a hand on his upper back. From 10 yards away, only body language could be made out when he began to talk. I saw the grieving husband register the cop's request for an alcohol test with no real facial expression. The husband looked extremely neutral, as if he knew that he was in for trouble — he appeared as if he was prepared to go to jail.

Watching the officer help the tear drenched husband up off the ground slowly, I turned to head for the ambulance — I needed to clear the stretcher of my medical bags and prepare for a blood draw. "Why did I have to be the paramedic on this call? Why did I have to be the jerk that does a blood draw on a guy who literally just lost the love of his life?" I thought. Talk about awkward... I've never been in a more awkward position in my entire life!

Moments later, the husband, who was being escorted by the facilitative cop, stepped into my ambulance. "Hello Sir, I'm Lorenzo. I'll be one of your paramedics for today. I've just gotta draw a bit of blood from you — we'll try to make this process as fast as possible. That's Jeff... He's my partner." The man looked at me with a dismantling gaze. I wasn't sure if he wanted to break down and cry or reach over and strangle me to death. What I do know is that his face was beet red with innumerable streams of tears running down his cheeks. He sniffled repeatedly, attempting to gather his breathing back to a normal rhythm. Jeff tore open the blood alcohol kit and handed it to me with vigor. It was understood that there had been a great tension the patient brought to our truck, one that needed great *relief*.

Neither of us wanted to be the ones who helped facilitate his going to jail if he ended up failing the blood alcohol test. We thought everything was taken care of after I vacuumed a few vials of blood from the gentleman — if only that were the case. By the time I completed the draws another on-scene cop poked his head inside the rear of the ambulance and said, "One more thing guys, we'll need you to do the blood draw with *our* police department blood alcohol kit. Protocol says we have to use the police department blood alcohol kit. It'll be another 30 minutes or so before an officer gets here with one because we keep them at our headquarters… Thanks" the officer said in conclusion and shut the rear ambulance door. "Wow… Really?!?" I thought to myself.

Jeff and I made friendly conversation with the man. He sat back, clasping his hands together in his lap. He stared off into the abyss for the majority of our awkward time together in the truck. Finally an officer poked his head in again with the new blood alcohol kit. Police had no more need for paramedic services after the task was completed. It turns out that the man went to jail for a DUI. Calls like this one are the kind that reminds me that this line of work includes not only good, but also the bad and the ugly. By now, one can conclude that a rippling effect of bad outcomes displayed on days such as this one is a reflection of the hideousness and ugliness the world of EMS can produce.

The Lord is good to those whose hope is in him, to the one who seeks him **Lamentations 3:25**

#40

Dad Crapped His Pants Again

***Paramedic Pointer*»** *Lift with your legs, not your back! Too many avoidable injuries occur in the work place from the lazy habit of bending at the waist to lift instead of allowing one's legs to do the work.*

Have you ever been to someone's home and thought, "It smells kind of strange in here?" Have you ever been to a person's house and thought, "Man, they need to clean up?" Yeah, well, some of the patients' houses paramedics respond to are downright horrific. Actually, I've got a better word for describing some of these homes: atrocious. Some of these people could care less about how their homes are contributing to their allergies and sickness. I've been in houses where hoarders live in a man-made maze. They leave just enough room to squeeze passed their piles and piles and piles of paper. Others simply don't clean up after themselves. There's a difference between hoarders and the messy; hoarders are organized in their messiness (if that makes any sense), they stack and categorize their piles of nonsense. Your average lazy person just leaves items strewn about with no order or organization to it.

Another standout house is the animal lover, the person whose house is a domesticated jungle for all sorts of critters. I've been to many different homes, but none (and I do mean none) could ever compare to the vile patheticness of one house in particular.

Responding to a traditional neighborhood home, Jeff and I paused for a second to review what the individual's chief complaint (reason for calling 911) was. "Oh boy, they gave us the generic *sick person* code" Jeff sighed. "Let's go and see what lies within this mystery," he said. Five minutes later we found ourselves outside an average looking house, parked directly underneath a streetlight. Dusk was falling rapidly; the street light flickered a few times before managing to shine brightly. There was a convenient sidewalk that ran from the street all the way up to the porch. Paramedics enjoy the conveniences presented to us such as this one because it means easy rolling for our stretcher wheels, as opposed to muscling our cot through grass or other rough terrain. We take what we can get with a smile.

KNOCK-KNOCK-KNOCK!! Jeff rapped on the residence door. "Paramedics! Paramedics!" Jeff yelled. Three seconds, or so, passed and a young blonde teenager answered the door. "Oh, hello... come on in," she said with a shy demeanor as she stepped to the side of the door. We brought our stretcher all the way inside the house. Paramedics learn quickly to get the stretcher as close to a patient as possible when the option is available. Many patients are not able to walk during their emergency. Some people are too injured, others are too sick. Then there's the group that is just too darn big to move themselves from one spot to the next, referred to in the medical field as the *bariatrics* category. There's nothing wrong with being a big individual, but when you're so big that you can't get out of your own way there's a problem. Beginning to ask where the patient was who called, I looked up and suddenly became mute by what I saw before me.

First of all, the scent of feces, urine and vomit mixed together almost caused me to faint! I thought to myself, "There's no use in becoming a patient Lorenzo, you'll only become an additional person for your partner and the next crew to deal with." I held my composure to the best of my ability, advancing toward the obvious patient, who sat comfortably in a filthy recliner. He was a Caucasian male, weighing easily 500 pounds. Trying to hold my breath, I asked, "What's wrong today, how can I help?" I'm now simply staring at a male patient who didn't even acknowledge my presence. "That's dad, he needs help," the teenage blonde who answered the door said. She was now sitting on a red couch with two other adolescents. Each of them was engrossed in the television show that was playing. Even the young blonde girl who spoke for her father talked to us while her eyes were glued to the TV.

"Does he have any medical history?" I candidly questioned her. "Yes, he's got high blood pressure. He crapped his pants two weeks ago… I think he did it again a few minutes before you all came," she explained in an eccentric, nonchalant manner. The other two adolescents were robotic in the way they carried out one motion: inserting their arms into a bag of chips and placing them into their mouths while remaining inattentive to their surroundings. I almost believed they were aliens. How can you choose to remain blissfully unaware of your own father who was rotting away in a *La-Z-Boy*? And let me tell you, that was a suitable name for both the chair *and* the patient! "When was the last time he's gotten out of that recliner?" I asked the blonde daughter of his. "He hasn't gotten up in two weeks or so," she murmured. "Wait, you said he crapped himself two weeks ago, you are telling me he didn't get up when that happened??" She nodded her head slowly, confirming that he did not get up when that occurred — not even to clean himself up. Accepting the conditions I was under, I asked Jeff to run out and grab our *patient mover*. The patient mover is pretty self-explanatory, only we use it primarily to move extremely large patients. Some paramedics refer to it as the shamoo/whale mover. Jeff returned quickly with our patient mover and two masks to help block the smell of rank feces. And thank God, because had it not been for that mask I don't think I would have made it!

Our goal when using this mover (which is basically a sheet with handles on the edges of it) is to stuff it under the patient completely so that they can become centered in the middle of it. So we began forcing the sheet under our patient as he sat in his recliner. Though he was wearing blue jeans, there was a nice pile of poop directly under him. His bowel movement must have seeped through his jeans with time and plenty of weight to push it through. "Got it! It's all the way under him!" Jeff gasped. Next we just needed to lift his legs up. They were no ordinary legs — these were the legs of a leathery skinned reptile, like a dinosaur. They had changed into an insanely tough, dark purple dinosaur texture. His toenails looked as if they had grown over the course of

100 years, they were sharp and long. I had to remind myself that I was indeed still dealing with a human being. Reinforcements showed up right when we needed them the most. A crew of firemen waltzed in and grabbed the handles on the patient mover. The dinosaur's… — I mean patient's vital signs were through the roof.

"Ready, set, lift!!!" commanded a large fireman. Three or four steps away our stretcher waited. PLOP!! Our patient landed safely on our cot — all *500 pounds* of him. "Let's go!" I prompted the team I now had. We performed a four-man lifting effort when we put the stretcher in the back of our rig. Jeff and I made eye contact once he was locked in; we were both struggling to remain conscious through the stench our patient emitted from his eroding body. "Waste no time Lorenzo, give that gas pedal your all!" Jeff said before he slammed the back doors shut from the inside the truck. It turns out that the bariatric (obese) patient was experiencing general weakness and a systemic infection… — with the way he cared for himself, I'll go as far as to say it's no wonder he hasn't died.

And they that know thy name will put their trust in thee: for thou, Lord, hast not forsaken them that seek thee. **Psalm 9:10**

#41

High Thresholds

Paramedic Pointer» *Flank (side) pain that moves to the posterior (specifically the lower back) is a hallmark sign of kidney stones.*

I was lucky enough to cross paths with a gentleman by the name of Luke. Luke had high standards. He was an engineer, educated at Yale throughout his college years. Luke ran his own engineering company; from what he told me, I gathered that he's a real overachiever. Jeff and I responded to a business building one afternoon to handle *flank pain,* as documented on our computer dispatch screen. Two feet beyond the welcome door lied a small office on the right-hand side. Behind a cherry wood desk sat Luke; he was leaned back such that all you can see from the doorway was Luke's head above an Apple laptop. Surprisingly, he stood up immediately when he realized we were the paramedics he requested.

"I'm happy you guys found us, we're kinda tucked away back here," he said, referring to his business' location. "With computer generated mapping systems, it's not too hard these days to find a place if you have the right address," I commented with a grin. "So what's going on today? Are you having some pain?" I inquired. A random voice shouted from the office across the hall, "He's alright! It's just Monday, so he needs an excuse to get out of the office." Luke laughed at the joke from a coworker and said, "My sides are hurting," pointing to both sides of his lower torso. "The pain moves around to my lower back area on both sides." "How long has the pain been going on for?" I asked. "Gosh, for about three hours now… I took some Advil expecting the pain to subside, but it only grew worse." "Well, the pain and locations you're describing are indicative of kidney stones, Luke." "Hmmm, that's odd… It doesn't feel as bad as my buddies have made out," Luke declared. He walked from behind his desk like his pain was totally absent. Sitting down on the stretcher, he said, "I usually just power through whatever aches and pains I experience until it goes away. I work out all the time — every day actually, so I'm sore all the time. But I must say, this is a bit different."

Luke was an extremely built man, muscular well beyond the average male — especially for someone his age. He looked to be about 40 years old. "How old are you Luke?" I asked him. "I'm 56 years old," he answered. "You look great for 56 years of age my man!" I complemented him. "Yep," he shook his head up and down with a big smirk. "I get up every morning to run 3 miles. I can do 50 pull-ups too," he said confidently. "Do you mean 50 pull-ups all at the same time?" "Absolutely" "You're not joking…you really are in great shape!" I blurted. "I like to set the bar high for myself in all areas of my life. Holding high standards has served me well," Luke said with satisfaction.

Upon locking the stretcher into the back of the ambulance, I then jumped inside to sit down on the bench seat. Slapping the blood pressure cuff on his muscular bicep, I said, "It's time to check out some basic numbers to get a baseline of where you're at." "Understood," Luke nodded. "Do whatever you need to do brother." As the blood pressure cuff inflated, I hooked Luke up to monitoring wires that would show the activity in his heart. "All vital signs look great Luke! Now all's we gotta do is juice you up with some pain medication so what would you prefer, a mild medication or one of my stronger meds?" "Oh don't bother brother, I'll be just fine…I can handle this," Luke explained. "You're going through kidney stones right now and you don't want any treatment for it?" "No thanks, it won't be necessary." "There's no shame in taking something to take the edge off," I encouraged Luke, sensing his efforts to be a tough guy.

"In fact, it's in my protocol to give pain meds to anyone who is having kidney stones… It's pretty much expected for the individual to need pain management… But hey, I can't force you Luke — it's your say-so in the end." "I really appreciate you, brother, I really do but I'm telling you, I can handle the pain," Luke replied. "Well, in that case, I won't draw up any drugs. The ER will want to draw blood from you, however, so after I start this IV in your arm, I'll leave you be." Luke cracked a smile in acknowledgment to my statement. "I must ask, though, how did you become such an ambitious man? What was it that sculpted you into the person you are today?" Luke gathered his thoughts, blinking continuously before opening his mouth to speak. "There's something beautiful about failure when you choose to turn it into creation. You know, as a young man growing up I failed a lot… And I mean it when I say a lot. Through all of my failing, I managed to develop discipline. Before I became ambitious and successful, I had no discipline. Some people refer to that lack of discipline as laziness, others call it resistance. Of all the things I enjoyed doing, engineering and physical fitness turned out to be my strongest areas, so I developed them both to the best of my ability and it paid off very nicely for me. I went from working for an engineering company to building my own practice — the building you just picked me up from. And with my development and working out, I now regularly attend competitions. They are lots of fun. So what I have learned is that through discipline you can be or do whatever you set your mind to," Luke concluded.

"That's pretty useful advice, thanks a lot for that Luke." "It's just the truth, if you got something you want to do, it then rests on your drawing up the blueprints of how to get there and executing!" Luke replied candidly. "Powerful, powerful lessons you're covering Luke, I appreciate it!" "No problem brother, just remember: people are their own worst enemy. Most of the time, the only person standing in the way is ourselves. No one can obstruct greatness from happening better than the individual themselves." "No doubt about that," I concurred. "Are we there yet?" Luke asked. Looking out of the window in the ambulance, I saw that we were about one minute from pulling into the ER parking lot. "Just about… We will be in 60 seconds or so." "Right on. Hopefully this process goes smoothly and quickly because I need to get back to work!"

For the Scripture saith, whosoever believeth on him shall not be ashamed. **Romans 10:11**

#42

Helium Heaven Or Helium Hell?

Paramedic Pointer» *A DNR (Do not resuscitate order) is a document that disables paramedics from making resuscitative efforts.*

On a cold, desolate afternoon when the city streets were drenched from the continuous pouring of rain, Jeff and I sat in the rig reflecting on some of the most ghastly calls our county has ever seen. A mysterious man was brought up who determined that his time here on earth had lapsed. A man who decided snuffing out his own candle would be the manner in which he checked out of this vast hotel stay we all refer to as life. To be perfectly clear and honest, this particular call was not a call I personally responded to. It is, nonetheless, a true tale from my county that I will tell in the first person.

Occupying lots of land stood an old two-story house. The abundance of land this house was surrounded by was farm-like, but there were no farm animals running around — there were no animals of any sort present on the property. The house looked to be built in the very early 1900s judging from the quality of the exterior and overall style of architecture. We were called to this location due to the 911 caller not having seen his neighbor in over a couple of weeks. An old dirt road led to this two-story house, which lied a ways from the main road used to navigate the municipality. A wooden swing, on metal chains, moved just barely with each wisp of wind. Approaching the old house, feelings of uneasiness invaded my mind. When you run enough calls, you sort of learn to pick up vibes that lead you to expect certain things. Things like *death*. The wooden swing creaked upon Jeff and I stepping foot onto the porch that rested above five stair steps.

A flyer of some sort was wedged between the screened in door at the entrance of the house. "What's that? An eviction notice?" Jeff joked. "It's just some restaurant advertisement," I replied while shaking my head at Jeff. KNOCK-KNOCK-KNOCK!!... "Paramedics! Is anyone here?!" I shouted. Peeking around the side of the porch, I saw an old Buick that had all sorts of rust build up on it. If I were to guess, I would guess that it wasn't operable. Pacing back over to the front door, I decided to twist the knob and push forward with my shoulder leaned against the door… the door was open. To my surprise, everything was neat and tidy — no evidence of a messy occupant, that's for sure. We both peered around the first floor of the residence as if our heads were on a swivel. "Maybe they're in the bathroom," Jeff whispered. "Why are you whispering?" I questioned Jeff as I took note of his troubled appearance. "Maybe they're in the bathroom," Jeff said once more in a normal volume, as if to prove that he wasn't freaked out. No one was in the bathroom on the first floor.

"Hellooooo…… Is anybody home?!" Jeff raised his voice. No response. "Let's check the patio in the back," Jeff suggested. We were on the hunt for a person who seemingly was not there. Advancing towards the patio to see if our alleged patient was out there, Jeff snarled, "I feel like were searching for a ghost." Nothing was on the patio except for an old newspaper. "Welp… the only place left to check is on the second floor of the residence; if someone is there, that's where they'll be," Jeff reasoned. From observing the kitchen area, a decently stocked pantry suggested that someone certainly lived here. Jeff and I started up the stairwell. "Who knows, maybe the person left town without saying anything," Jeff reasoned. "Like a vacation, you mean?" "Yes, not everyone tells their neighbors when they are going to be gone for a few days. I sure don't anyway, my neighbors are creepers! They'd probably break in my house and steal from me if they were certain I would be gone for a while!" Jeff explained. At the top of the staircase, a cracked doorway allowed the stream of light to shine through. Dust particles danced in the beam of light shining down on the staircase from the doorway. It made me aware of all the crap I was breathing in.

Arriving at the doorway, Jeff and I made eye contact before moving forward through the door, we both knew something wasn't right — and we were about to find out exactly what that was. "Here goes," I said to my partner Jeff with one hand resting on the center of the door. I slowly pushed it forward. The next thing that appeared before our eyes was unnerving. Next to a queen sized bed (which was perfectly made up) sat a person in a rocking chair with a brown paper bag over their head. Clear tubing ran from inside the paper bag down to what looked like a metal oxygen tank. Inching closer to the patient, the tank had the word *helium* ingrained in the metal tank. Also, there were a stack of boxes neatly placed on the floor about 5 feet in front of the victim. They were labeled, interestingly enough. Each had a person's name on the box. One had *Sarah* written on it. Other names included *Sam, Tony, Jessica, Tim...* There were about 15 boxes total. Just a foot or two away from the victim was a small ottoman. A small piece of paper rested delicately atop the ottoman with instructional notes numbered one through nine. "These are directions for how to properly perform suicide by way of helium induction," Jeff said, as if he had been trying to decode a mystery. "Yeah... I heard about this before... people claim this to be a moderately peaceful way to commit suicide because it's non-invasive, as opposed to hanging oneself or shooting oneself." "I'm not so sure any form of suicide would be peaceful, Jeff" I stated. "Well if you think about it, you're not really even suffocating yourself. You're displacing the oxygen in your body and replacing it with helium... you end up getting so high off of the helium that you end up passing out and stop breathing inadvertently.

All the while, your unconscious so the person just kind of sails away." "You seem to know about this as if you've done it firsthand, Jeff, are you sure you haven't tried this and failed?" I cut my eye at him facetiously. "Hahaha no, I have not attempted to do this, I just happen to know a thing or two about it. But I gotta say, he planned this thing out well. He's got everything boxed up and labeled. Apparently he knew what family members he wanted each of his belongings to go to," Jeff said with an impressed look on his face. We had not taken the brown paper bag off of the man's head yet, but the rest of the body clearly showed that it was a male we were dealing with — an abnormally hairy male at that. When Jeff pulled the brown bag from over the victim's head, an excessively long bearded male was underneath. He had turned ghost white.

The clear tubing was taped to his cheek, running right into his mouth. His body was extremely stiff, from head to toe. His arms that rested naturally on the rocking chair's arms were nearly immovable due to the stiffness. He wore a brown flannel long sleeve shirt rolled up to his elbows. He also had on blue jeans and brown boots. Our victim was DOA (dead on arrival). His body had not decayed yet, but the rigor mortis (hardening of the body) had set in for sure. "Hook him up to our cables to capture an asystole (flat line) waveform for documentation," I directed Jeff. Jeff tore open a package of cardiac electrodes to put on the victim's body. I looked around the room, wondering what pushed him over the edge. What could have been so bad in this person's life that he rationalized taking his own life? There were no signs of a wife or kids — no picture frames or female jewelry stands. I went into the closet and there looked only to be men's clothing. I thought there may be a suicide note/letter that he left behind. His last words, so to speak. But no letter was left behind. All there was as far as any writing was the directions he scribbled down on a piece of paper from a website.

"All done!" announced Jeff, unhooking the cables from the victim's body. It's too bad that we didn't show up in time to talk him out of going through with suicide. Calls like this forced me to wonder what our victim believed in, if anything. The funny part about death is that no man or woman has come back from death to speak of what is on the other side. You can't ask your late grandmother or grandfather what lies on the other side when one dies. No. That's against the rules. You must believe that something great awaits you, and that requires none other than *faith*. I'm not sure where you stand right now as far as faith, but I believe that if you accept Jesus into your heart that you will be saved. Not necessarily saved from the tragedies of this world, but from longsuffering in the eternal realm. If you suffer from depression, suicidal thoughts, or general confusion about why you're living, try Jesus on for size, he might fit.

For I will restore health unto thee, and I will heal thee of thy wounds, saith the Lord. **Jeremiah 30:17**

#43

My Insides Are Going To Explode!

Paramedic Pointer» *Factors contributing to pancreatitis (inflammation of the pancreas) include increased alcohol consumption, medication reactions, trauma, cancer and gallstones.*

Sometimes an acute emergency can arise so abruptly that you have to drop everything you're doing — literally. A construction worker building a new school allegedly dropped the ladder he was carrying and the bag of tools in his other hand. It was a member of a construction team who was known for his punctuality, hard work and tenacious demeanor. It is individuals such as this fella who make one say, "Nothing can keep him down!" And on a typical day with no X factors, that statement would be right more often than not. But today was different for this hardworking citizen. My partner Jeff and I responded to a walk-in clinic for reported *chest pain* and *abdominal pain.* About seven people sat casually in the waiting lobby while faint grimaces and groans echoed somewhere in the rear of the medical office. Though these grimaces and groans were faint, they were indeed audible, but no one so much as fidgeted from the newspaper they were reading or the cell phone game they were interacting with.

"Can someone let the paramedics back here!?" The front desk attendant screamed impatiently. "I'm on an important call with the state!" The brunette female explained. No one answered her call and no one appeared. Jeff and I waited in the lobby to be let through the doors that led to the patient evaluation rooms. 20 seconds or so passed on by before the petite, brunette female rolled her eyes and said, "Can you please hold for just one moment?" on the telephone, realizing that no one was near the front end of the clinic to assist her in helping us through the doors separating the main lobby from the private evaluation rooms. She frantically pressed the hold button on her telephone unit and slammed the phone down on to the receiver. Using both hands to push up from her desk, she nearly lifted off of the ground when she got up to let us through the door. "I'm so sorry guys," she said apologetically upon opening the cherry wood partition door. She put the back of her hand on her forehead, looking as if she wanted to convey the body language that is seen when someone is hot. Her acrylic nails, a bright pink color, had neat little flowers on them. "Your patient will be down the hall in the first door to your right when you turn the corner," she explained in an emotionally drained fashion. "Thank you," Jeff and I said one after another as we fled down the hallway. "Oh my God!!" an anonymous man's voice crescendoed the further Jeff and I advanced down the corridor. "What in the world is happening to me?!" the unknown voice rang out once more. We turned the corner upon reaching the dead end of the corridor and saw a wide open door. Our patient was sitting on an evaluation table, shirtless, covered in cardiac electrodes (cardiac stickers, simply put). On the righthand side of the room stood a white coat (slang for a physician/doctor) that immediately turned towards us when he heard our steps.

"Hello gentlemen, this is Roger. I have just evaluated his heart and he is experiencing a heart attack. He also has excruciating abdominal pain in all quadrants of his abdomen. He was working on a construction site when the sudden onset of pain came on. Roger is 59 years of age," the doctor finished. "Hook Roger up to our cardiac monitor once we get him seated on our stretcher," I directed Jeff. "Sure thing, okay Mr. Roger... I'm going to square the stretcher up right next to you so all you have to do is scoot over, no standing necessary," Jeff instructed. "There we are," Jeff said once our cot was perfectly placed to transition Roger from the evaluation table to the cot.

"Now give me about three big scoots so that you're centered on our gurney," he instructed further. Roger gave 1 ½ scoots, seemingly giving out of energy. He sat there with beads of sweat accumulating on his forehead. The physician, myself and Jeff instantly stepped towards Roger as if he had a magnet pulling us toward his body.

Grabbing under each of his armpits, we slid him over to the stretcher in one motion. Jeff began to yank out the cardiac wires to hook Roger up to our monitor. "When did this pain start, Sir?" I asked. "When I was at work on the construction site," Roger replied. In Roger's lap rested a lime green construction vest with reflectors on it. (Those reflectors come in handy, as well as the bright neon green. Drivers just don't seem to pay attention, so the more obvious you can make yourself while working by traffic the better). "Can you describe the quality of the pain — "AAAHHHHHHHH!" Roger interrupted with a painful shriek. "I think my insides are going to explode!" He screamed under a tremendous amount of pain. "Where exactly do you feel the pain, Roger?" I quickly responded to his beckoning bellow of pain. "Everywhere! It's mainly in my chest and my stomach," the 59-year-old caucasian construction worker grimaced. "I'm gonna need you to stay nice and still for about 20 seconds or so, Roger, we're going to take a snapshot of your heart so we have a picture of it from our own equipment" (the walk-in clinic had already taken an EKG prior to arrival).

This was probably the last thing on earth Roger wanted to hear. Sit still? While I'm in the worst pain of my life? "What an ignorant request," Roger must have thought in the midst of his devastating discomfort. And to make matters worse in terms of my request, I also asked him not to speak or make a peep to the best of his ability. I know, I know. It sounds harsh. But trust me, it's completely necessary. Fidgeting, shaking and any noise made from a patient can greatly alter the quality of that cardiac snapshot we capture. It's imperative that there is minimal artifact (false readings) on the printout we assess. Discerning whether someone is having a heart attack or not is no careless task. Roger did an immaculate job sitting still in spite of his current condition. The cardiac printout slowly unraveled from our monitor. I tore the paper away and held it taut for a clean read.

"That's a heart attack alright," I thought to myself. Keying up my radio mic, I advised, "I've got a STEMI alert!" (Medical terminology for heart attack). By now it was confirmed twice that Roger was in bad shape. Jeff, grasping the foot-end of the cot and I the head-end, we raced for our truck. With no time to waste, Jeff and I blitzed Roger with *oxygen, nitroglycerin, aspirin and morphine*. "Let's get out of here…now!" I frantically told Jeff. "You got it, we'll be transporting emergency," Jeff said in his deep voice. Transporting emergency means with lights and sirens on the way to the ER. "Am I gonna make it?!" Roger asked me with a desperate look of hope in his crystal blue eyes. "We're doing everything we can to help you. When we get to the hospital, it's going to then become a matter of getting you up to the Cardiac Cath Lab," I explained. "You guys are great… really. Thank you for all your help," Roger said with his left hand holding his chest. He then became silent and slowly closed his eyes, trying to find peace in the midst of chaos.

"Don't close your eyes, I need you to stay awake for me Roger," I urged him. "Alright, aright" he reluctantly replied. Minutes later we found ourselves busting through the ER doors with a team of nurses ready for action. Transfer of care was made once we got Roger up to the Cardiac Cath Lab. As we usually do, we followed up on Roger a couple days later. Roger had a few cardiac stents placed. He managed to survive the brutal heart attack. Oh, and it turns out his torso was intact — in other words, his insides didn't explode.

*And ye shall serve the Lord your God, and he shall bless thy bread, and by water; and I will take sickness away from the midst of thee. **Exodus 23:25***

#44

Potential To Drown In One's Own Fluid

Paramedic Pointer» *Congestive Heart Failure (CHF) is a cardiac condition where one side of the heart is overworked, resulting in fluid backing up into the lungs. These patients experience severe breathing difficulty, as you might imagine.*

We've heard of the cliché drownings. People have drowned at sea, in the pool, lakes etc. All of these are indeed tragic. I'd like to introduce an *uncommon* way people drown. I'm not the kind of person to mention problems without at least being willing to solve the problem, so by the end of this tale, we will have covered the solution. Drowning in your own internal fluids is a problem if there ever was one. "How on God's green earth could someone drown in their own fluid?" you might ask. It's called CHF, short for *congestive heart failure*. What happens, in short, is a person's blood gets backed up in the chambers of their heart — so much that it backs up into the lungs.

Your two lungs are reservoirs for air. When those reservoirs get filled up with fluid, we begin to suffocate. Because, as we all know, humans don't breathe anything but air, unless of course you're a mermaid or merman. Have you ever tried to breathe in underwater? If so, you ended choking and had to come up for air. But on the flipside, we know that there is no issue in breathing *out* while underwater. This is how congestive heart failure works. Patients experiencing CHF typically find it difficult to get air *into* their lungs but don't have much difficulty getting air *out*. But all the while, their lungs are slowly filling up with fluid, taking up more and more of their ability to breathe.

Imagine that actor on the movie who's trapped in a room that's being flooded to the ceiling, you can envision them holding their mouth up to the ceiling as they float atop a room full of water slowly consuming them. That is essentially what's going on with the CHF patient, only it's going on *inside* their body, specifically their lungs. With that being said, you'll never believe the positive spirit one patient was in while in this particular condition. Not only was he all smiles, but he was cracking jokes! My partner Jeff and I responded to a Caucasian male named Charles. He was in an apartment on the second floor. There were only stairs leading up to the second floor — no elevators. For this reason, we brought our stair chair, a piece of equipment used to move patients down staircases. It's much too dangerous to attempt hauling the stretcher up and down stairs without a patient on it, let alone with a person sitting on it! I could see a door chalked wide open in making it to the top of the staircase. Blatant clues such as doors wide open, houses being the only one with lights on in the middle of the night, and sometimes even a person waving the ambulance down make finding a patient much easier for paramedics.

Stepping into the patient's apartment unit, he quickly became visible — he sat upright on his couch with both hands on his knees. He was leaned over and working hard to breathe. Firemen, who were on scene already, had placed him on an oxygen mask, but it didn't seem to help. Have you ever blown bubbles in your soda as a child? (Lord help you if you still do and you're an adult). The bubbly sound heard when one does that is exactly how Charles, our patient, sounded. The bubbly sound, as you might imagine, grew louder and louder as Jeff and I inched closer to the Caucasian male.

I started to take my stethoscope from around my neck to gather lung sounds, but they were audible already. For some odd reason, Charles was filled with glee. No, he wasn't mentally challenged or psychologically imbalanced. It turns out, according to his wife, that Charles found a way to crack a joke under any circumstance. "Oh Charles, you are a handful," the wife said referring to Charles' preparing to cut up. "Are you fellas sure you know what you're doing? No one's going to give me mouth-to-mouth are they?" Charles joked. Though odd, it was refreshing to see a patient in such good spirits in the midst of a potentially life-ending occurrence such as CHF. "Take it easy on me, whatever you do; at 68 years old, I'm not what I used to be," Charles said with a gleeful smirk. "How long has it been since your breathing difficulty began?" I questioned. "Don't make me think about it, this has been a problem of mine for over 10 years— and running! As you can see," Charles said.

Assessing his pulse oximetry (a device that measures how much oxygen is in your blood) the reading was dangerously low. "Get him on a breathing treatment — fast!!" I directed. "Put him on our CPAP machine," I specified. An example of how the CPAP machine works is when you roll down the window speeding down the interstate and open your mouth outside the car. There's massive amounts of air that enters one's mouth — the CPAP machine affects one in the same way. After all, CPAP stands for *continuous positive airway pressure*; no one who has taken the highway wind speeds directly in their mouth can deny that it is definitely continuous when it comes to airway pressure! "You may have seen this already (CPAP machine) and know how it works, Charles, but don't be alarmed at the air pressure… breathe it in as well as you can," I coached while helping placing the device on his face.

"Oh no… not the master blaster!" Charles chuckled. "Okay," he said, confirming that he understood the procedure. A fireman whipped the coffee table out of the way because it was right in front of the couch Charles was sitting on. We placed our stair chair precisely in front of Charles so that all he needed to do was stand and pivot onto the chair. "We're going to have you stand and sit right back down, Charles," I informed him. He gave me a big smile, though he was severely under distress, and proceeded to maneuver onto the stair chair. Charles was sweating his butt off, breathing heavily, and had a slight purple tent to his face, indicating his breathing distress. CLICK-CLICK-CLICK! A fireman and myself buckled Charles into the chair and began towards the stairs just outside the doorway.

His oxygen saturation began to rise substantially — he was improving! What happens is all that air pressure forces the fluid out of his lungs. Another way we evacuate fluids out of a patient's system is with a drug called Bumex — Bumex causes you to urinate. In cases such as these, where a person is suffering from excessive fluid, I'm sure you can calculate the value removing fluid has. Once again, another unstable patient turned into a stable patient once Jeff and I intervened. Charles improved more and more on the way to the hospital. When we administered *Nitro*, another useful drug for CHF, Charles improved even more! In a sink or swim predicament, Charles was able to stay afloat, so to speak, above and beyond his own internal fluids.

In the house of the righteous is much treasure: but in the revenues of the wicked is trouble. **Proverbs 15:6**

#45

Unexpected Station Visit

Paramedic Pointer» Maintain situational awareness in every environment. Be prepared and expect the unexpected. Preplanning is where success really happens.

Every now and again paramedics receive an unexpected visitor who waltzes right up to our quarters and rings the doorbell. It happened this time around our lunch hour. My partner and I were planted firmly in our chairs, pulled up unnecessarily close to the dining room table. My partner Jeff was enjoying spaghetti; I was devouring a plate of chicken and vegetables when the automated visitor notification interrupted us —"ATTENTION! YOU HAVE A VISITOR AT THE OFFICE FRONT DOOR," the electronic woman advised us over the intercom. I heard Jeff gulp one last wad of spaghetti down in a hurry as he stood up; I wiped my mouth clean, following closely behind him out the dining room door. We paced expediently across the ambulance bay (garage for ambulances) to the opposite side of our station.

Opening our front office door, we were presented with an elderly lady with super dark shades on. "It's Ralph, he's acting very strange... *unusually* strange. He's been stuck in the same position for about 10 minutes now. This isn't normal for him!" The elderly woman cried. "What kind of position are we talking about?" I asked the woman. "He's got his right arm held up, pointing his index finger straightforward!" She explained under deep anxiety. Over to the right in our small parking lot was a small SUV parked facing the station. It was an extremely bright day out. At this point, I gathered the woman's reasoning for her super dark shades.

Sure enough, an elderly gentleman occupied the front passenger seat just as his wife described — to the tee. He gazed forward — his mouth halfway open as if he were awestruck by one of the *seven wonders of the world*. Had you taken a glance at him, you'd have thought he actually saw something that totally blew his mind. But this wasn't the case at all. There was only our station before him — and there's nothing mind blowing about an EMS station. "What's going on today, Sir," I asked the man. He seemed to be frozen in place. "What are you pointing at Sir?" I asked the older gentleman. No answer. "Can you hear me Sir?" I questioned him. Again no answer. Turning around to face his wife I asked, "Is this normal for him to not talk?" "No, no not at all, he talks all the time. He was just talking to me when I was driving along. He stopped speaking in mid-sentence." When he didn't respond I panicked and came straight here.

"What do his vital signs look like, Jeff? I asked. "Not too hot... his blood pressure is through the roof!" he replied. "When was he last seen normal?" I asked his wife. "How long *exactly*? Was it when he suddenly stopped speaking mid-sentence?" "About 25 minutes ago," the patient's wife exclaimed. "Jeff, is he weak on either side of his body? Can he follow any commands?" "Other than his right arm and hand being stiff, he's weak everywhere else. He cannot follow commands — that is a negative. "Let's get him packaged up on our cot, I'm calling a stroke alert." Changing tac channels on my mic before keying up, I advised, "Medic 16 has a patient with stroke-like symptoms; this will be a stroke alert."

"Copy medic 16, at 1530." Ralph's right hand was almost immovable. When trying to intentionally reposition his arm, it was too stiff. Jeff even forcefully pushed it downward and Ralph's arm sprang back up like a slot machine lever in Las Vegas. Thinking about what was before my eyes almost became comical in my mind. Here's a guy who is pointing forward with an intensified gaze in his eyes — strange, to say the least! Even though situations can be found humorous, we paramedics do our best to remain professional.

I'm asked all the time when sharing stories with friends: "Were you able to keep a straight face when...?" I always tell them the same thing, "As much as I want to crack up, I keep it professional" — and I do. I've come across some of the most outrageous things that would have one rolling on the floor with laughter. As nice as it would be to burst into tear-producing laughter, it's simply not a good look.

The chances of a patient being offended are much too high — that's the last thing one would want from a paramedic who was there to make things *better*. Transporting Ralph gave me a new definition to the phrase *frozen in time*. Ralph didn't budge the entire ride to the ER. His vital signs remained ridiculously high as well. Evaluation at the hospital gave the staff a flummoxed outlook on his stiffened right side. Other than this unknown reaction, all signs were indicative of a stroke: altered mental status, high blood pressure and neurological deficits (weakness). Expediting Ralph up to the CT scan room, a physician met us outside, anxious to get Ralph on to the evaluation table. After moving him over to be scanned, a technician said, "I need everyone out of the room so that there's no interference in capturing the patient's head scan!" Hearing this, Jeff and I exited swiftly.

And this is the confidence that we have in him, that, if we ask anything according to his will, he heareth us: and if we know that he hears us, whatsoever we ask, we know that we have the petitions that we desired of him. **1 John 5:14 – 15**

#46

Prayer For Healing

Paramedic Pointer» ***Fracture*** *= broken bone,* ***Sprain*** *= stretching or tearing of a "ligament"(usually leads to swelling),* ***Strain*** *= stretching or tearing of a "muscle" due to overuse.*

As a believer in Christ, it's important for me to extend the message of faith to you. Faith is believing in something you *can't* see. Faith is the hope one has that something will happen that they believe to be true. Many great things can be accomplished when one has faith, because before something happens, an individual must first *believe*. Faith is present in our everyday lives, we just don't think about it. We have to have faith that drivers will stay in their lanes when we're cruising down the street. We have to have faith our restaurants won't poison our food when we dine out.

We have to have faith that our fellow paramedic or nurse will not harm us intentionally when it's help that we need. Faith is everywhere! And it is faith in God that will ultimately save your soul and your life eternally. It won't be the doctor's great skills. It won't be the paramedic. It won't be the fireman or policeman. What's going to save you — and yes I'm talking to you, reader, is faith in Jesus Christ — that he died for your sins. Accept him into your heart and you'll never regret it, especially on the *Day of Judgment*, the day when you and I's good deeds will not suffice. We will be judged based on whether or not we know Jesus Christ — God's son.

A call I responded to one afternoon gave me great joy. Jeff and I responded to a church located in a small community called *The Christian Retreat.* As you may imagine, it had been a Sunday morning, church service had just let out. A slew of people poured out of the church doors, migrating towards the parking lot. Though the rumblings of numerous attendants flying out of the church made great noise, a "crack" brought all of the rumblings to a startling silent pause. A woman was down. This is when someone phoned 911 because we had been dispatched to "A woman down… possible ankle fracture."

Upon entering *The Christian Retreat* community, we saw a crowd of people gathered in one spot. "That must be where our patient is," Jeff proclaimed. Pulling closely up to this group of people, we both observed that everyone — who by the way, were fully dressed up in church attire, had their heads down. "What are they doing?" Jeff questioned. In addition to everyone hanging their heads down, each one of them also had their eyes closed. "They are praying," I answered. "Oh… okay, that makes sense," Jeff reasoned. Their whispering prayers were audible just as I opened the passenger side door to step out onto the black pavement. It was a charming sight to see. No one had any medical equipment to assist the downed patient physically, so they took it upon themselves to assist the uninjured woman spiritually.

"OOOHHH JESUS! OOOOHHH JESUS! PLEASE MIGHTY GOD!!! HEAL ME LORD!!! GIVE ME THE STRENGTH LORD!!!" She cried. "What happened to her?" I asked a man who looked to be the head pastor. I quickly knelt down next to him, at her side, so that I could hear him despite the surrounding noise of the woman crying loudly and the adamant prayer warriors. "She was walking out to her car just like the rest of us and tripped over the speedbump!" he said leaning in closely towards my ear. We were straddling a generic speedbump — the annoying yellow ones strategically placed in parking lots to keep one at bay.

"Gather some supplies to splint this ankle!" I called to Jeff, who was already walking towards me with the cot. He made a quick turn to race back to the truck for more equipment. Our patient had to be over 300 pounds, easily. This told me that there was an awful amount of pressure coming down on her ankle once she tripped over the yellow speed hump. Her *open* ankle fracture explained just how much pressure on her ankle was involved. Blood dripped generously from the left ankle fracture, onto the black pavement. If you've ever held an ink pen firmly on a piece of paper, you'd find that the pen consistently bleeds out, causing the initial dot you made larger and larger. The same result can be achieved with coloring markers. This was the precise effect the female patient's droplets of blood had on the concrete due to dripping repeatedly in the same spot.

"Excuse me sir," Jeff said as he stepped in between the pastor and I to immobilize the open fracture. "I'll hold it steady if you want to do the bandaging," I said to Jeff. "Absolutely, let's make this fast so we can move her onto the cot," he replied. It took about one minute or so to successfully bandage the woman's ankle. No bleeding seeped through the bandage either, not all the way at least. Jeff used plenty of gauze pads to absorb the blood. The white cotton bandaging became a faint red, but nothing too excessive. "We're gonna roll you onto this backboard in a few seconds," I advised the heavy woman. To properly move her, we needed to first get her onto something rigid. "ONE… TWO…THREE…ROLL!" I shouted. Jeff and I slid the long spine board under her once she was resting on her side. "…ANNDD BACK DOWN!" I instructed.

Getting all 300+ pounds of her centered took a bit of effort — to say the least. Jeff took the foot of the backboard while I positioned myself at the head-end. "Ready when you are!" I shouted to Jeff. We were both squatting in preparation to lift our patient up and onto our stretcher. "READY…SET… LIFT!" Jeff chanted.

Our next priority was getting some potent narcotics into her system to alleviate the pain. Zooming over to the rear of the ambulance, Jeff and I performed a double lift to lock our patient in place in the rear of the truck. "Set up an IV for me Jeff!" I directed. "What's your name miss?" I asked our patient. "I'm Lorenzo, and he is Jeff… we will be helping you feel better this Sunday morning the best we can, okay?" "OOHHH JESUS! OHH JESUS!…UHH… I'M ANGELA! Thank you for your help guys! OHHH JESUS LORD HELP

MEEE!" "Not too much longer now, Angela, I'm drawing you up some mor-phine as we speak." "OOHHH PLEEEASE HURRY!" The female patient cried in agony. I juiced her up with a generous dose. "We can get going, Jeff," I prompted. In checking Angela's vital signs, they weren't doing bad at all. "What is your pain on a scale of 1 to 10, 10 being the worst pain you've ever felt in your life?" "OOHHH JESUS AT LEAST A 12!" Angela shrieked. Noting her great distress, I began drying up a dosage of Dilaudid. Angela needed something with more *kick* to it.

I speedily screwed my loaded syringe into my IV access point. With no time to lollygag, I pushed the medication into her bloodstream. "AAHHH.... THAT'S MUCH BETTER...THANK THE LORD," Angela exhaled with satisfaction just moments following the administration. "What is your pain scale *now* Miss Angela?" I inquired. Taking a deep breath and exhaling again, she answered, "IT'S TOLERABLE NOW...NOT COMPLETELY BETTER...I'D GIVE IT A 5 OUT OF 10."

"Very good. We'll be at the ER in no time okay... then the Doc can check you out further." "CAN YOU GET ME A WARM BLANKET PLEASE... MY BODY IS COLD!" Angela stated. "Absolutely," I replied, as we sailed on down the busy street.

The Lord shall cause fine enemies that rise up against thee to be smitten before thy face: they shall come out against thee one way, and flee before thee seven ways. ***Deuteronomy 28:7***

#47

Miracle Miss

Paramedic Pointer» *If a pregnant woman has sustained trauma and is bleeding massively, the maternal circulation will shunt blood away from fetal circulation to maintain maternal homeostasis—maternal circulation takes precedence over the requirements of the fetus.*

How do you determine a miracle? When I think about a miracle, I wonder, "What are the specific guidelines?" Is it something that has to be universally agreed upon to be deemed *miraculous*? One pastor defined find a miracle in a sermon I saw as an *unsolvable problem that becomes solved*. He was ministering to the congregation on how to receive a miracle from God. His instructions were to present God with a problem you can't solve (unsolvable problem) and if God decides to solve it for you, then you've received a miracle from God. Other individuals, perhaps, see miracles as fictional... a mere expression of the English language synonymous with the phrase, "that's unbelievable!"

Then there are those of us who are on the fence about things such as miracles. Things are said like, "That had to be a miracle... but then again, it could've been a fluke... things could've lined up by chance." The Bible speaks of miracles. As an avid believer in Christ, I believe that miracles are real.

Further, I believe other kinds of divine intervention is very much alive today too. This tale reveals a very unlikely outcome for a pregnant female who could have lost her life. Whether her fortune was a miracle or not— I'm not sure— I'll leave that up for you to decide.

Late one night in the tumultuous zone 16, a woman, age 22, called 911. The byproduct of her calling for an ambulance generated a pop-up on my ambulance computer screen disclosing that a black female patient was wounded. "Light it up!" I urged Jeff from the passenger seat. His head was leaned up against his window and he had just begun drooling from the corner of his mouth — he was sleeping. Jeff tried to adjust himself like he was slowly waking up, only his eyes never opened. I took my eyes off of him, thinking he was waking up to get a move on, but soon realized this was not the case. I looked over at him once more and found him to be slouched down with his cheek against the driver side window yet again.

Shaking my head, I said, "Jeff! Light it up! It's time to go!" "What? Huh?!" Jeff mumbled, waking up with brief confusion. It was 1:30 AM or so, and to Jeff's credit we had already ran the gamut on emergency calls throughout the day. He had every reason to be tired. Emerging quickly from his disorientation, Jeff wiped his mouth and sat upright, placing his foot on the gas pedal. "I'll route you on the way to the call," I said, just before we raced down the street. Five minutes later, Jeff and I found ourselves in the heart of the ghetto. The neighborhood was quiet for the most part, just an occasional lowlife walking by on the sidewalk grasping a bottle of vodka.

Now in the vicinity of our call location, we turned the sirens off so that we wouldn't wake the neighborhood. We kept our emergency lights on, however, and crept slowly past a few blocks until we saw police lights about halfway down one block. Talking to a police officer in the front lawn of a residence stood a young black female who was clearly pregnant; in fact, she looked as if she was going to burst! Jeff and I said to one another, "She may be wounded, but she's walking wounded!" An oriented, independently standing patient is always a positive sign in a paramedic's eyes. The young black woman seemed to be doing fine, her body language conveyed a surprisingly calm demeanor. "Good evening gentlemen, this is Tamika," the police officer greeted us. Tamika gave a broken smile and a partial wave. She was only about 120 pounds. "Miss Tamika has been shot three times, but fortunately, they only grazed her body.

"I've seen bullets graze the skin before, but not three times on the same person — someone must be watching over you…" he said, turning towards Tamika. "… A guardian angel." The policeman started to cough heavily — a smoker's cough. Catching his bearings, he turned up his face and said, "What kind of an idiot would shoot at a helpless pregnant woman anyway? I mean seriously?"

"Are you able to take a couple steps to our stretcher, Tamika?" I asked her. Tamika looked at me and slowly shook her head up and down just enough to communicate a yes. "Come on over and take a seat right up here," I said, pointing to the upper end of my cot. She sat down very carefully and I asked her, "Where exactly are the bullet wounds?" "Two are on my back and one is on my thigh." I lifted up the backside of her shirt to quickly assess the wounds holding a small flashlight in my hand. About 8 inches apart were two small circular wounds with fresh blood resting inside of them. I then shined my flashlight on her thigh and a similar wound was located on her quadricep. "How are you feeling? You seem to be painless just looking at you," I stated. "Ummm…" Tamika began, "I'm not in much pain at all, mostly shell-shocked," she replied. Jeff and I placed her inside the rig for further evaluation. CLICK-CLICK!! I flipped on the dome lights, illuminating the rear of the rig (where we perform patient care).

Reevaluating her wounds once more, it was mind-boggling that the bullets didn't actually pierce her flesh. "How did you end up getting shot at?" I inquired. "It was a drive-by," she began. "I was walking outside of my house, back and forth on the phone, when a random car drove by and started shooting!" Tamika explained. "Does someone have it out for you…an enemy maybe?" "No, I don't think anyone I know would do this," Tamika said softly. "The officer was right… Someone must be watching over you." "I think so too," she said calmly. "These small wounds technically won't even need any bandaging because they're not actively bleeding!" I told her in astonishment. "What we're going to do, though, is start an IV on you so that we have access to your body. Your vital signs are immaculate; everything else looks good as well." Pressing down gently around each bullet wound, I felt for a possible bullet beneath her tissue that may have been overlooked. All clear. I couldn't believe it. It was a privilege to have witnessed such a patient.

"We're gonna transport you to the trauma center in the nearest hospital," I advised Tamika. "No more guns or bullets from this point forward, only a smooth ride to the ER." "Okay," Tamika replied with a smile of relief.

What a near miss event! Statistically speaking, the percentage of individuals having dodged three bullets all at once has got to be next to impossible! The only person I've known to dodge bullets was a fictional character named Neo from a movie called *The Matrix*. The call was rare, and almost impossible it seems, but it was anything but fictional. Tamika, in a way, had dodged bullets. Her fortune was, by any person's definition, unbelievable.

But I will deliver thee in that day, saith the Lord: and thou shalt not be given into the hand of the men of whom thou art afraid. For I will surely deliver thee, and thou shalt not fall by the sword, but thy life shall be for a prey unto thee: because thou hast put thy trust in me, saith the Lord. **Jeremiah 39:17 – 18**

#48

Vampire Suicide

Paramedic Pointer» *No breathing and no pulse warrants the need for CPR to be initiated in most situations. Push hard and fast in the center of the chest after calling 911. Remember to lock your elbows. (google or youtube "Lorenzo Hogans II-How To Do CPR" for a fun video)*

People commit suicide in various ways. My partner Jeff and I reflected on crazy calls that the county of Manatee has hosted. Hangings, drug overdoses, blasting one's head open with a shotgun, jumping off of bridges and asphyxiation via creative methods are some of the ways people go about taking their own lives. One call came up in our conversation that could very well top all of the suicides in terms of *peculiarity*. This tale is an emergency response that I was not in attendance of. What I will do, since the tale itself is 100% true, is tell it as if I were there; it will be told, as are all of my tales, in the first person. Shall we begin?

Progressing into the latter portion of our 24 hour shift quite nicely, the clock had just turned 9:42 PM on Wednesday night. *Possible Suicide* was the pre-arrival notes provided to Jeff and I from dispatch. Little did we know what we would be walking into. Statistically speaking, suicide was most popular on Wednesday for some reason. My college sociology course required students to do a paper on the matter. I can't remember too many of the details, but I do recall that suicide is more prevalent in males because of the assigned responsibility from society on the male to be a sole provider. More specifically, the white male held the highest suicide numbers of all.

"But why Wednesday?" My sociology teacher candidly asked on that particular day. Everyone raised their hand, including me. "What do you think the reason behind Wednesday is, Mr. Hogans?" my professor called on me. "I think people are having trouble finishing off the week and rationalize it better to pull the plug, so to speak, on themselves than to endure the rest of their week." My professor responded with an acknowledging "Hmm" and continued gathering answers from other students in the classroom. Once he finished taking answers, he revealed that I happened to be correct.

There was a majestic mansion out in Lakewood Ranch, Florida— this is where our victim resided. Outside in the driveway was a bright red Lamborghini. The Lamborghini was parked on the left side of the half circle driveway, tilted upward slightly on an incline. "We'll have to be careful not to hit that in passing," Jeff said almost drooling over the automobile. "Snap out of it, Jeff," I said sarcastically. Just after Jeff and I pulled our stretcher out of the back of the Ambo, a fire engine pulled up behind us. Three firemen jumped out with Halligans and flat headed axes for forcibly entering locked doors.

"We were told there might be trouble trying to get in," one fireman informed us. Approaching the front doors, which had a large glass panel one could see through from the roadside, everyone's demeanor changed. About two weeks worth of newspapers were piled up in the semicircle driveway, likely the clue that a neighbor took upon themselves to initiate a welfare check. When you see someone every so often and it abruptly ceases, suspicion begins to set in. It's nice to know that there are people who genuinely care about others' well beings in this day and age. It was a good thing the fireman already came with tools in hand because it saved them a trip back to their fire apparatus. We found out moments later that the door was locked — it would need to be pried open.

"One – two – three" BOOM! "One – two – three" BOOM! "One – two – three" BOOM-POP! The door flung open, revealing an awfully large, vacant first floor. Walking into the mansion suddenly made the five of us reduce to the size of ants in proportion to the vast establishment. "We'll check the second floor while you guys check down here," I said, referring to Jeff and I searching upstairs. "Wow… this place is made of money!" Jeff whispered to me as we paced up the stairwell. No one was to be found in the upstairs bathroom. Two of the three second floor bedrooms were empty as well. At the end of the hallway lied the final room — there was a crack in the door. "If there's no one in here, then this place must be empty," Jeff said to me. Pushing the door forward, we heard a yell come from downstairs.

"No one is on the first floor! We checked everywhere!" A fireman shouted. Both Jeff and I stood in awe of the sight directly before us. A man lied on the bed — clearly lifeless. "Eeeyeah…he's up here… the patient is up here… we found him!" Jeff yelled back. Neither of us budged upon realizing the eccentric picture placed before us. Lying on the bed was a man who resembled a vampire — to the tee. He wore a tuxedo — all black with a bright red tie. His hair was slicked back with what must have been three full bottles of hair gel. The Caucasian male victim's mouth rested halfway open, exposing vampire fangs that overlapped his lower lip in the corners of his mouth. But that's not it — a wooden stake was lodged in the man's chest on his left side — right where his heart was. And to put the icing on the cake in terms of creepiness, the entire room was lined in plastic!

So we stood there attempting to make sense of it all in our minds. "What the…" a voice suddenly broke the uncomfortable silence. The three firemen had just made it upstairs to partake in the observation of a seemingly supernatural fatality. Had we not known that vampires were fake, we would have easily been fooled. This particular fellow was made up perfectly to fit the mold of a bloodsucker. How he managed to thrust a wooden stake into his heart — I don't know. As much money as this guy had, I wouldn't be surprised if he paid someone else to kill him — especially when you consider how he allegedly drove the steak into himself with that much force!

However he did it is a wonder to me. One thing for sure is that he had a keen interest in vampires. From his red Lamborghini to his slicked back hair and fangs — he indeed died *as* a vampire—or at least the closest thing to it. Due to only seeing this man when he died, it causes one's mind to ponder if he tried to live as a vampire on a day-to-day basis. All indicators of a person being dead were present: line of lividity, rigor mortis, no pulse/breathing and last but not least, cold to the touch. There was no bringing this fella back. Not today.

But the Lord your God ye shall fear; and he shall deliver you out of the hand of all your enemies. **2 Kings 17:39**

#49

I Can't Go To Jail!

Paramedic Pointer» *The normal respiration rate for an adult is 12-20 breaths per minute.*

I t's never a good thing when you end up at the wrong place at the wrong time. But we, as individuals, couldn't possibly control these kinds of variables — variables such as timing. No one has the ability to permanently rid themselves of misfortune; if they did, half of the EMS calls that are generated wouldn't exist. On the positive side of this inevitable truth (our lack of control over timing and misfortune), a safety net has been put into place. Emergency medical services is that safety net, we are the helping hand that picks up individuals in need. We are the restoration squad who responds to restore the balance. It is for this reason that I decided to switch lanes, so to speak, in college.

I originally was going to pursue a degree in business management, but turned to EMS after my freshman year. The thrill of action drew me in. Whereas, sitting in a cubicle pushing a pen over monotonous documents for 20+ years didn't sound too enticing. But helping a person when they are sick or injured rang a bell in my brain. I thought it purposeful to be a man who mends things that are broken, a voice of reason in times of struggle. We paramedics are present for the good times, certainly the bad times and yes, even the downright ugly times. Here is a portrait of one of those ugly times, the kind of times you don't really want to look at because you simply don't have an award-winning solution for it.

At about 3 AM, an accident occurred just before a bridge heading towards the beach. Jeff and I knew there were two people involved— at least— because our notes generated by dispatch disclosed that it was a vehicle versus a bicycle. Both Jeff and I were clothed in our nighttime jumpsuits. "Make sure you remember to put on your traffic vest," Jeff cautiously reinforced. We were crossing a narrow, narrow bridge where all one could see clearly were the reflectors on the road for the most part. Glancing briefly to the left and to the right, I saw the sparkling shimmer from the moon reflecting off of the miniature waves in the sea — it was a dark, still night. Up ahead were the entrancing police lights pulled over on the shoulder of the road.

Over in the grassy area aside from the road, an officer perused the bushes with a flashlight, it appeared that someone or something was lost. Once aware that our ambulance had made it on scene, the officer suddenly turned around, blinding us with his LED flashlight. That flashlight was as bright as can be, as all officer flashlights seem to be. They must have a standard they go by when purchasing flashlights: MUST BE ABLE TO CAUSE INSTANT BLINDNESS. The policeman began to jog back towards our unit while we stepped out of our tall front cab.

"Hey guys, we've got a vehicle versus a bicycle… the driver of the vehicle looks to be intact, he's still in his car. Your other patient is a man as well, but… he's not doing so hot. He's right over in that area," he said as he turned and made circles on a bushy area with his flashlight. Jeff and I made haste to go and evaluate the unconscious man. Unconscious turned out to be an underestimation. From the time we came into a close enough distance to make out anything visible, it became evident that the gentleman's head was submerged in blood. I saw no rise and fall of the chest (an indicator of a breathing patient). His neck looked to be broken. "This guy really took a blow," Jeff stated. Kneeling down to assess our patient's neck, I felt nothing. Feeling the back of his head felt like gory mush — he was *long* gone.

He was a victim of what we call unsurvivable trauma — there was no need for resuscitation for him because there was zero chance of him regaining life. Sometimes paramedics do what is referred to as a *show code*. This is when a paramedic still goes through with an elaborated attempt to resuscitate a patient when he or she knowingly has no chance to successfully revive the person. It happens normally when family is present so that they see that everything that could have been done was carried out for their loved one. It shows that the paramedics genuinely tried — hence the name *show code* (code means cardiac arrest).

KSSSHHHH! "Medic 16, we have two patients on scene, one is dead on arrival," I spoke into my portable radio. Pacing over to our other patient in the driver seat of his vehicle, we could see the young man crying relentlessly. I leaned over, inches next to his rolled down window and asked, "Do you have pain anywhere?" "I've got a little bit of lower back pain and I feel like there's a bunch of glass in my mouth." "Open up, say ahhh," I instructed him. He opened his mouth wide; I could see small grains of glass everywhere. There were small pieces of glass stuck in his bottom lip too. I opened his car door and stepped inside to look at him a bit closer. "Would you like to go and get checked out at the ER?"

"WHERE'S THAT OTHER GUY? IS HE OKAY?!" "Don't worry about him right now, you are our concern." "WHERE IS HE?! IS HE OKAY?! I NEED TO KNOW!" the patient cried. "IS HE OKAY?! —I HIT HIM!—I DIDN'T SEE HIM…HE WAS RIDING HIS BIKE IN THE MIDDLE OF THE ROAD!" "Do me a favor and just try to calm down for a minute okay… what is your name, for starters?" "Rashad! My name is Rashad!!" Rashad resembled Bob Marley, only the mulatto version. He had long black dreads and a mustache just like him. "Let's get you into my ambulance for transport," I recommended. Frustrated, Rashad hung his head down and followed me into the rig — he was well enough to walk. Once I realized that he was on the verge of a panic attack, I figured I better get him into the ambulance before I told him the outcome of the guy he ran over.

After the final buckle clicked on his seatbelt straps, Rashad urged me to tell him how the other patient faired. "IS HE OKAY? YOU HAVE TO TELL ME MAN! I'M FREAKING OUT HERE!" Reading my face before I even opened my mouth, he blurted, "OH NO…IS THAT GUY DEAD??" "Yes,"

I answered. "YOU'VE GOTTA BE KIDDING ME! MY LIFE IS OVER! LOOK AT ME! I CAN'T GO TO JAIL! I'M GONNA SPEND THE REST OF MY LIFE GETTING RAPED! AS SOON AS I WALK INTO THE COURT ROOM THE JUDGE IS GONNA TAKE ONE LOOK AT ME AND SAY, "PUT HIM AWAY!" I'M A MINORITY MAN! AND LOOK AT ALL THESE TATTOOS I'VE GOT! MAN, IM DONE!" He cried. "AND I'VE GOT CHARGES FROM MY PAST! I JUST MOVED DOWN HERE TO BE WITH MY WIFE AND DAUGHTER FROM BALTIMORE! I'M FINISHED!" He concluded.

"Don't be so hard on yourself, brother. Your fate has not been sealed yet." "YOU DON'T GET IT! I'M THROUGH! WHAT WAS THAT GUY EVEN THINKING?! IT'S PITCH BLACK OUT HERE AND HE'S RIDING IN THE MIDDLE OF THE ROAD!" He continued to cry. "Like I said, don't throw in the towel on yourself just yet, accidents happen and people are aware of that. Trust me, I see genuine accidents all the time." "ALRIGHT MAN... I'M DONE WHINING...I'M SORRY." "I understand how you feel, trust me. No need to be sorry. Just try and keep a level head for now — no sense in getting yourself all wound up until you know what's what. Rashad maintained stable vital signs for the duration of the transport. He was more shook up than anything else. I patched him up where needed before arriving to the ER, which primarily involved removing all of the tiny glass particles engorged in his bottom lip.

Ye that love the Lord, hate evil: he preserveth the souls of his saints; he delivereth them out of the hand of the wicked.
Psalm 97:10

#50

I'll Jump!

Paramedic Pointer» *Veins carry deoxygenated blood to the heart. Arteries carry oxygenated blood away from the heart; the exception being the pulmonary arteries (carries blood to the lungs for oxygenation) and pulmonary veins (carries oxygenated blood).*

Having a gigantic bridge in my district of duty created an eye-opening revelation to me — people are committing suicide multiple times a week. Connecting Pinellas County to Manatee County is a famous bridge called the *Skyway*. Whenever it came up in conversation, if my dad was around, he would tell you of how it collapsed years ago; how it was so dark and foggy for people who were driving over the edge, plummeting down to their death unexpectedly. Since the collapse years ago, there has been no unexpected free falls by individuals utilizing this particular bridge — keyword *unexpected*.

Rather, people are doing it on their own via suicide attempts. For this reason, there has been two red phones issued on both northbound and southbound lanes of the *Skyway*. If you are to cross the bridge, you would see them up there, placed in the center of the bridge where the highest point is. If you ever decide to give suicide a go, just remember, it's never too late to phone in a voice of reason.

It has been said that there are generally two outcomes on Skyway suicides — death and death. But the manner in which you die is contingent upon where one hits. "There are two ways people die," said one fireman who'd been on countless responses to the gigantic bridge. "People hit the water, break every bone in their body, and drowned to death… and then there's those who hit the rocks and die on impact… — Aim for the rocks is my advice."

At first it amazed me that I hadn't heard of the innumerable suicides performed from the Skyway, but then it dawned on me that the news stations would be reporting the same story almost every other day. I mean seriously, how would that 100th suicide report be conveyed? "Reporting *again* on suicide… another Joe blow decided to jump again today to his death." Also, how would that affect citizens living nearby? It may scare them into moving someplace else — the city wouldn't necessarily want that would they? Or maybe even worse than citizens getting freaked out, what if they all kinda just got desensitized? It happens all the time with the youth via video games.

One Skyway suicide attempt stood out from the rest. It is a tale that I will tell in the first person as if I were there. Nonetheless, it is a true tale that should be told. Early morning, just 30 minutes before our 7 AM shift change, the emergency bells alarmed all of us. "Possible suicide" is what the automated female's voice said over the intercom. The fire truck responded with the ambulance for good measure. Zooming towards the Skyway, our unit tilted back slightly as our front tires made contact with the foot of the incline on the vast bridge. Driving up the Skyway is always a thrill because it's so darn tall! It has these huge golden beams that glisten in the sun. If you stare straight into the sky as you travel up the incline, you'd feel as though you were ascending into heaven.

Nearing the tip top of the intimidatingly tall bridge, there on the right side was a man in a business suit standing on the edge. He was holding a briefcase; his long red tie flapped in the wind. Cars passed by, creating gusts of wind that I feared were going to tip him over before any of us could rationalize with him. We exited our emergency vehicles after we parked a considerable distance away from the potential victim. Easing towards him slowly, we all began to speak at once… "Sir, we're here to help you, just think about what you're doing here, okay?"

"LEAVE ME ALONE! The man barked. I CAME UP HERE TO DIE AND THAT'S WHATS GOING TO HAPPEN!" "I understand Sir," Rich said, a fireman. "But think about this for a second Sir, I reasoned with the patient. There's no sense in doing this," I continued. "I TOLD YOU THAT I WANNA DIE! I CAN'T TAKE THIS ANYMORE!" "Sir," Richard started —"DON'T COME ANY CLOSER!! I'LL JUMP!"— Jeff, myself and the three firemen all stopped dead in our tracks. We were only a couple of paces away from the jumper. The man standing on the edge slowly turned his head toward the ocean and stared out into the distance, taking his eyes off of us. Standing close to the edge myself, I leaned over slightly to see what looked like a bottomless pit of fog. The fog was so thick that virtually nothing could be seen beyond 5 feet or so down below.

The jumper adjusted his stance, scooting just a tad bit further onto the bridge's edge. He squatted, ever so slightly, creating a bend in his knees that was barely discernible. As the Caucasian male jumper prepared to launch himself from the edge, Rich sprinted towards him. You would have thought Richard was a track and field Olympian the way he dipped his head downward and propelled himself forward with a sleek stride. Just as the jumper's fancy business shoes lifted about 1 inch from the edge, Rich arm-tackled him and landed with him on the pavement. The look on the jumper's face was one of both disbelief and discomfort. The two remaining firemen, along with Jeff and myself, ran over to Richard and the jumper. Richard was lying on his stomach with one arm wrapped tightly around the jumper's midsection.

"Well done Richard," one fireman applauded him. "Great job," Jeff and I followed. The jumper, who was laying on his back, slowly lifted his head to get a look at us all, but let it drop back down to the pavement in an instant. Richard winced. He acquired multiple abrasions all over his muscular fore-arms. Police units pulled up so close that it seemed they were trying to ride up the back of our heels. Two policemen hopped out with horrified looks on each of their faces. There's something called a Baker act that warrants an individual to be held in custody if they want to harm themselves or others. Normally it results in the person being taken to a crazy house. The two policemen slapped a pair of handcuffs on the jumper once Richard rolled off of the Caucasian male. Before 60 seconds passed, the Caucasian man was escorted into the back of the police unit.

That the blessing of Abraham might come on the Gentiles through Jesus Christ; that we might receive the promise of the Spirit through faith. **Galatians 3:14**

#51

Guns & Fire

Paramedic Pointer» *Always put your safety first if deciding to help others in distress. There's no benefit to creating additional patients. (Example: violent or belligerent people, unsafe environment, negative intuition about anything)*

As if a fully involved structure fire wasn't enough, add a gunman to worry about shooting himself or shooting you. At 1 AM, the tones went off. "STRUCTURE FIRE! STRUCTURE FIRE! STRUCTURE FIRE!" That's the luxury of this line of work (I say that sarcastically). No matter what you're doing, when the bells ring, you are leaving whatever you're doing — fast. I happened to be tucked away under the comforter in my station bed this time around. I had just fallen sound asleep too, but duty superseded my desire to stay in bed.

We nearly rode on two wheels when we bent the first corner leaving the station. Jeff was really psyched for this call once he found out that there was both a house on fire and a man walking the premises with a handgun. I guess he equated the added threat of a gunman to mean excitement. I'm not exactly sure why, especially when that gunman could point a gun at us! The call location was no more than three minutes away — we arrived in no time. Let me tell you, the flames engulfing the house were absolutely radiant. We saw nothing but yellowish orange flames swallowing the house with no remorse. Firemen were already on scene, but they were fighting the fire from across the street.

"Why would they be fighting the fire from across the street?!" You might ask. Well, because of the crazy man with a gun walking around in the backyard waving it around. As firemen, they had a duty to put the fire out, but personal safety comes first in all matters. Police were on scene, but this was a mission they felt more suitable for the S.W.A.T. team. So we waited halfway down the street because of the alarming safety hazards before us. The man waving the gun around could very well shoot someone; there was no sense in putting ourselves in danger.

An abundance of water was shot on to the house, but with no effectiveness. The very end of the water stream was all that made contact with the house, which resulted in the fire only receiving a light sprinkle. "Do you think he's going to off himself?" I asked Jeff while we waited patiently in the silent cab of the ambulance. "How long have we been here now?" He answered my question with a question. "About 20 minutes or so." "No," Jeff answered. "You know how these things usually go Hogans, people who wait this long don't usually go through with it," he finished. "Yeah you're probably right." I saw a shadow race across the yard directly across the street from the house fully involved with fire. Suddenly I saw another dark shadow. And another one. I managed to catch the lettering on the next dark shadow. In bright white bold letters I read: S-W-A-T.

The Special Forces had arrived and were already in motion. Jeff and I rolled down our windows anticipating the sound of gunshots. No gunshots yet. What we did hear, however, was the voice of the homeowner making threats to everyone. "DON'T COME BACK HERE! I MEAN IT! I'LL SHOOT!" he yelled violently. We drove up closer to the house so that we'd be ready to intervene where needed. Just moments after we repositioned the ambulance, I noticed two S.W.A.T. soldiers creeping across the street into the gunner's backyard. "IF ANYONE COMES BACK HERE I'LL SH..." —POP-POP-POP-POP-POP!!! The S.W.A.T. soldiers moved in on the crazy man under the cloak of darkness and shadows. Not to mention, their all black suits contributed to blending in with the night. KSSHHHH! "The scene is now stabilized... paramedics, you can move in!" A man's voice notified us over the radio. We came to find that the gentleman was very much... alive. The S.W.A.T. soldiers shot him a total of five times — one bullet in every limb, but one limb had two bullets.

"This guy is dead," a firefighter/paramedic said rashly. "Oh wait, I was wrong — he's got a pulse and breathing!" he corrected himself. Jeff and I rushed in, beginning to control bleeding from each of the bullet holes. The patient's eyes opened, looking around in an overwhelmed onslaught of fear. "IT'S SOOOO PAINFUL!!" The downed gunman winced. His verbal complaint let me know that he had a patent airway. This was a positive thing to me; it meant that I wouldn't have to place a breathing tube down his throat to manually oxygenate him.

Placing him in the rear of the ambulance, Jeff and I started IVs in both of the gunman's arms. Putting fluid bags in place, they swung from the ceilings during each corner we turned. "It will only be a few minutes before we get you to the hospital Sir!" I advised. "AAHHHHH! THE PAIN HURTS SO BADD!" the now gunless man cried. Jeff handed me a dose of fentanyl to administer. "This ought to ease the pain a bit!" I stated while pushing the medication into his vein. "I SURE HOPE SO! IT HURTS TERRIBLY BAD!" he grimaced. His vital signs were a bit out of whack, but you'd expect that to be the case when a person has been shot five times. Everything happened so fast; just a few seconds ago our patient was marching around his backyard making threats with a firearm — now he lay on his back with blood leaking through the holes in his body. We managed to maintain a viable blood pressure en route to the ER. Our gunman probably didn't suspect that *he* would be the one getting gunned down. From the looks of things, our patient would be okay; he just needed to get those hot bullets removed from his limbs. What a wild night it was, but with it now only being 2:15 AM, we still had five hours left to go until shift change — go figure.

And every man that hath his hope in Him purifieth himself, even as he is pure. ***1 John 3:3***

#52

Seizing The Moment

Paramedic Pointer» *Following a seizure, patients often go through a phase termed postictal. This is where they are aphasic (unable to speak), confused or unable to follow commands, very emotional, and tired or sleepy. Gradually the brain will begin to function normally.*

There isn't one designated reason for seizures, there never has been. In pediatric patients, there is what's called febrile seizures, or seizures caused by *fevers*. In pregnant women there is a condition called *eclampsia*, where a pregnant woman's blood pressure rises so high that she begins to seize. Other seizures result from chemical imbalances in the brain. There are so many different ways a seizure comes about. We've all seen them occur in one way or the next, whether on television or our cousin who was flopping like a fish on the bathroom floor. I don't suppose there has ever been a right time to have a seizure, but how about experiencing a seizure in the middle of a fight? It's not like having to go pee or suddenly getting the hiccups. No, your coherence is absent! Your movement is uncontrolled. And oh yeah, you are likely to have trouble catching your breath because you can't breathe!

In an apartment complex located in zone 16, timing couldn't have been worse. Leo was throwing down on his neighborhood rival. Shirts off and fists up, subsequent blows were dealt amongst the two fighters. Except that one blow — a blow so traumatic that it sent Leo into a full-body seizure, that's when the restoration team showed up (i.e. Jeff and I). "MY BABY! MY BABY...! MY BABY IS HAVING A SEIZURE! HELP HIM!!" A random black woman in scrubs ran up to the truck as we slowed to a complete stop. BANG-BANG-BANG! She knocked on the passenger side window with a bawled fist, urging us to make haste in helping her son. I motioned her to back away from the ambulance so that I could open my door without knocking her down. She reluctantly backed away with both hands covering her mouth. In walking fast to the rear of the truck, I noticed that Leo had handcuffs on. He was lying on the concrete with his legs propped up in a police unit as if he just fell out of the officer's backseat. His light hazel eyes were widened with disbelief.

Though he appeared aware of the internal imbalances that caused his body to quake, he had no control of the constant twitching. Jeff and I each opened one of the rear ambulance doors at the same time to pull the cot. The worrisome mother, who had followed me step for step, cried "IS HE GONNA BE OKAY? PLEASE TELL ME HE'S GONNA BE OKAY!" I turned to her, just before we pounced on Leo, and assured her, "My partner and I are going to do everything we possibly can." She stood back at this point, content with my word. "So what exactly was he doing when the seizure started?" I asked the on scene officer. "This young man instigated a physical altercation with another teen male here in the complex, they were fighting one another when he began to seize." Leo, still actively seizing, shook violently from head to toe. He looked like a worm that had electricity running through its body. "Pull the stretcher right up next to him," I directed Jeff. "You ready to lift him up?" I asked my partner. "Whenever you are," Jeff replied. "And... Up!" I shouted, as we secured Leo in our grips.

In one fluid motion, we elevated him and lowered him gently on our cot. "Let's roll!" I said as we made a team effort to wheel him on our stretcher to the ambulance. Upon locking him into place in the back of the rig, Leo's seizures stopped. Leo was winded; his whole body was limp with weakness. He was in a phase referred to as postictal, a state of disorientation and weakness directly following a seizure. "Can you hear me Leo?" I asked him. With a hanging, drowsy head he mustered up enough energy to open his hazel eyes and look at me. His eyes were such a light hazel that they gave off a penetrating gaze. I waited for a response. Nothing came. —BLAAAHHHHH!—Leo vomited; it tumbled down his chin and fell down onto his bare chest. Leo looked down slowly to try and register what just happened. He began to dry heave, yoking his head back and forth. "Get me a vomit bag for him!" I urged Jeff, who was sitting next to the cabinet they were kept in. Right before Leo upchucked a second time, Jeff had already torn open the packaging and held the vomit basin below Leo's mouth. —BLAAHHHH! — Our patient barfed again — this time a longer-lasting spout of throw up.

Grabbing towels from a compartment sealed by a sliding glass door, I cleaned Leo up — the vomit was everywhere. I started an IV to administer fluids. "Uh-oh! Do you have some Ativan prepared? Because we're going to need it! Leo looks like he's starting to seize again!" Jeff warned. When I looked up from finishing the IV, Leo began to twitch. Immediately, I leaned over him to take out our medication box from the cabinet above. "Ativan… Ativan… Where are you?" I thought calmly to myself. It's not that I didn't know where it was, it was the fact that the 33 drugs we use had become mixed around in our medication box, making the Ativan a bit harder to find. "There you are!" I thought to myself after sifting quickly to find it.

As quickly as I could, I hooked up the now loaded syringe to my established IV access point. "Pushing the initial dose of Ativan," I verbalized to Jeff, who sat with our toughbook (laptop for patient reports) in his lap. He documented the time of administration right on the spot. Monitoring Leo for a change, I sat back and observed for a few moments. To our satisfaction, the Ativan had worked! For a second time, Leo came out of the seizure completely gassed. His entire body looked drained of energy, which isn't out of the ordinary for a seizure patient. "Welcome back once again, Leo," I greeted him. He tried intently to focus his eyes on my face, but had minimal luck. It looked as if his efforts to focus on anything only made him dizzy.

"Quick prick in your finger, Leo," I advised him before sticking his index finger. My intentions behind pricking him was to collect a droplet of blood from my glucometer; Leo's blood sugar needed to be assessed. When a person has a long seizure or multiple seizures, all of the violent convuslions burn up the sugar in one's body. Leo's blood sugar turned out to be well below normal limits. "Prepare an ampule of D50," I asked of Jeff. Jeff held the loaded ampule over at me to take from him. Leo's low blood sugar contributed to his disorientation, it was too low to function normally. "Almost there," I said aloud as I neared the end of the ampule. Fully pushing the last bit of the ampule in marked an increase in mental status for Leo.

He began blinking constantly, regaining the alertness he once had. "Are you back with me?" I said with a gentle smile. "Where am I?" Leo asked in a daze. "You're in the back of an ambulance— you had a seizure. We gave you some anti-convulsive medication for your seizure and some liquid sugar because your blood sugar was low. "… Oh… thanks…" he whispered. "The hospital is going to do some blood work on you when we get to the ER. Just relax and enjoy the ride for now." Leo looked down and around, realizing that he vomited all over himself. "When did you do this?" He held up his arm to show his IV. "While you weren't very alert," I answered with a slight smirk. Leo gave no response, as he was trying to make sense of all that was before him. This was a day to remember — or *not* remember in Leo's case. Even though he had been in a fight, put in handcuffs, had a seizure, vomited and suffered altered mental status, these happenings never happened as far as Leo was concerned.

For the hope which is laid up for you in heaven, whereof ye heard before in the word of the truth of the gospel. **Colossians 1:5**

#53

Crossing At The Wrong Time

Paramedic Pointer» *Look both ways before crossing the road. Even though pedestrians have the right of way, always be defensive when it comes to traffic, whether walking or in a vehicle.*

You'd like to have one of the buttons at every intersection with the light up man who lets you know when to cross the street or stay put. Every intersection can't necessarily employ the system, but it would be nice. That particular system is interwoven with the traffic lights — meaning the light up man isn't going to signal you to go if there is through traffic speeding passed due to a green light. That's the beauty of technology, it relieves some of the workload, focus and overall energy we have to expend.

At 11 PM or so on a Monday night, one 10-year-old boy didn't have the luxury of the pedestrian crossing technology at the intersection he wanted to cross. He had to use his own judgment — no big deal — it's not as if he was a toddler or anything; he had good sense. But sometimes it's not always about the judgment and attentiveness of the pedestrian, even if they are as young as the fellow I'm getting ready to tell about. Jeff and I snapped our neon green traffic vests together as soon as we got word that a pediatric patient was struck by an automobile. To our surprise, the call did not come from zone 16 (our zone of duty and also the busiest zone in the county of Manatee). We were summoned to cover for another unit who was already tending to a different emergency response.

Located on a freeway style intersection, Jeff and I cruised down the road going about 65 mph. Up ahead, we would soon see revolving red and blue lights coming from on scene police units and fire apparatus. "Start slowing down," I suggested to Jeff, "with there being so many units on scene, we'll let the fireman controlling traffic direct us where he prefers us to park." In the center of the intersection sat a boy on the grassy median. His hair was jet black, he wore a gray hoodie. Built pretty stocky, the boy looked to be rather chubby. He was surrounded by EMS and police department personnel. Jeff and I bypassed pulling our cot out of the ambulance because we opted to get a handle on the gravity of the emergency first — our young boy looked to be ambulatory (able to walk).

"Excuse me… excuse me," I said, trying to make my way through a few cops and firemen to evaluate the young boy. "What is your name?" I asked. Whimpering, the boy said, "Jo Jo". Tears cascaded down his face, he was filled with anxiety. "Would you like to tell me how you got those scratches all over your face?" He had abrasions taking up half of his face, distributed in different spots. Sniffling, the young Hispanic boy began, "Yes… I was standing on that side of the road," he pointed behind me, "And I began to cross the street… I thought the car was going to slow down but-but-but they never diiiiddd!" he stuttered. "So did you get knocked down? How did you get these scrapes all over your face?" Still sniffling with anxiety, he said, "The car hit me and I rolled over the top of it!" He explained through a snotty nose.

"WHERE'S MY DADDY! I WANT MY DADDYYYY!" —Out of the cluster of personnel on scene appeared a Hispanic man wearing black slacks and a navy blue polo shirt. "Jojo! Jojoooo! Oh my goodness Jojo, are you okay buddy?!" Sniffling profusely, Jojo said, "EEYEEESSS!" crying a river after forcing out his response to daddy. "Jojo, I need you to tell me everywhere you feel pain. You can point to it as well so I know exactly where you hurt." "My neck hurts a little bit, my back, my chest and my ffaaaaccceeee," he cried with more sniffles. "Okay well what we're going to do is take you inside our ambulance and put on what's called a C collar to stop your neck from being able to move around. It's important we protect your neck considering the fact that you were just hit by a moving vehicle okay Jojo? And by the way, my name is

Lorenzo, but you can call me Lolo if you want. That's my nickname. It rhymes with yours."

I extended my hand to Jojo to help him up from the curb. "Will I be okay Sir?" Jojo asked me while walking behind me towards the truck. Turning around briefly to make eye contact, I began to snicker a bit, "Right now you're a walkie-talkie and that's one of the best signs that you're going to be okay." "A wha…?" Jojo muttered. "Hahaha, a walkie-talkie, it's what paramedics refer to people as that are able to *walk and talk* on their own — walkie-talkies!" Letting Jojo step up into the ambulance from the sliding door on the side of the truck, he asked, "Do walkie-talkies get needles??" Jojo stood frozen, looking up at me with hopeful eyes in anticipation for my reply. "No… Not this time around buddy, you've got nothing to worry about!" Sliding the door shut behind us, we both took our seats — he on the stretcher and I on the bench seat. It was a wonder that Jojo managed to get away with just superficial scrapes. No broken bones, no busted organs or nerve damage beset him. In a match of boy versus machine, Jojo walked away with minimal battle scars — I would deem him the winner.

Whosoever therefore shall humble himself as this little child, the same is greatest in the kingdom of heaven. **Matthew 18:4**

#54

Ah-choo...A Baby!

> **Paramedic Pointer»** *Contractions that are more than 5 minutes apart generally mean you have time to take a pregnant woman to a nearby hospital. Contractions less than 2 minutes apart signify an imminent delivery!*

Medical professionals don't deliver babies — women do. Rather, we assist and facilitate the birthing process to the best of our abilities. I don't want to take any of the credit owed to mothers who struggle and fight through that God awful pain of conceiving. And I believe I speak for all medical professionals when I say to all the mothers, "The credit is all yours in delivering babies." I consider it a true blessing to have helped with two deliveries thus far. It's not every day a paramedic responds to a pregnant woman during the short window of imminent delivery — it's all about timing. In fact, some paramedics flaunt it among other paramedics when they assist in these calls because it's a rare occurrence.

True story: I was texting one of my paramedic buddies about something random, it was mainly general *catching up* type conversation because we had not communicated in over a year. We were firing text messages back and forth like bullets. I found it interesting that he never responded after I text him, "You'll never believe it! I just assisted my second childbirth man!" He's been a paramedic longer than me and I'm almost positive he hasn't assisted even one childbirth, so I hope it didn't bother him. But the funny thing about this particular call is that what they say about the higher count of deliveries a woman has under her belt, the faster the next one will be, is true! I found out firsthand.

Jeff, my main partner, called out on this shift (which he later regretted). A real fireball named Ashley occupied Jeff's seat in the ambulance today. To give you a snapshot of what Ashley was like, picture a pale blue-eyed redhead with pasty white skin. She sort of resembled Mary Jane from *Spiderman* in appearance, only no where near as serene. She lived on caffeine — didn't matter if it was coffee, Mountain Dew or what have you. I believe she had some pent up anxiety issues because on the way to this call she was blasting the air horn excessively, and I mean every bit of it when I say excessively! HONK-HONK-HONK-HOOOOONNKK!! "These idiots need to move it! What are they, senile?!" she would yell. Ashley came off as one of those people who "nut up" when they gain a position of authority.

Our computer screen populated the location we were responding to on the map. It also generated our call notes that were put in by dispatch. "Imminent delivery… delivery number four" is what our screen showed, that is all we had to work with— and the fact that our patient was 22 years old. "My goodness," I thought to myself on the way to the call. "We've got a hot little something on our hands" I said to myself while trying to figure out what age she must have started having babies. "I've got the child birthing kit," I told Ashley as we exited the truck. We brought a few extra bags inside in case of an in-house delivery, leaving our stretcher fully packed with equipment.

Grandma was sewing on the couch as we rushed inside; she didn't get startled one bit. On the floor were the patient's three children, playing with toys and wrestling. It was night and day— the living room in comparison with the back bedroom— where mommy was. It's amazing how two rooms, literally right next to one another can have such opposite vibes! The living room harbored innocent joy and carelessness — an environment of leisure. Mommy's bedroom held a tension so great that you could have cut it with a scalpel. Mommy was lying down on her bed with a black T-shirt on, naked from the waist down. She was a small Hispanic woman, no more than 120 pounds. "This is Maria, she's pregnant with her fourth child... she's having contractions lasting for 30 seconds at a time, we need to make a decision — like now — whether to try and transport her or set up for delivery." "How often are the contractions occurring in frequency?" I inquired. "About seven minutes apart." "We are only six minutes or so from the nearest hospital, let's get a move on to transport her!" I urged.

"NOOOO, PLEASE DON'T LIFT ME!!" The Hispanic woman begged. She was in a tremendous amount of pain, as you may imagine. "Sorry dear, but we have to move you... we'll be as quick and as gentle as we possibly can," said one fireman. "AAHHHHH!" the small woman cried as two firemen effortlessly cradled her and placed her softly on our cot. Rolling vigorously over the tile floor in the hallway outside the bedroom, Maria let out another long cry, "AAHHH!" she screamed. Ashley took a peek under the white sheet we draped over Maria's bent knees, her eyes became huge. "Her water just broke!" Ashley announced. When we passed the living room, one of the toddlers looked up and said, "Bye-bye mommy", waving slowly with his miniature hand while sitting crisscross applesauce. With a patient in a predicament such as this one, expediting transport was a decision that went without being said. Ashley made sure a fireman rode along with her in the back of the ambulance; as for me, no later than I slammed the driver side door did I wait to apply foot to gas pedal.

"Take it easy on us Lorenzo! We're gonna be back here standing the whole time!" Ashley shouted from the rear. She was referring to the fact that she didn't want to be knocked over during transport. The movement in the rear of the truck is about 10 times as much as the front cab. I took the corner slow, using straightaways to accumulate good speed. "We're pulling in now!" I yelled to Ashley and the fireman performing patient care in the back. Our mission was to get Maria up to the labor and delivery department before it became too late. Time ticked against us — every second counted. A hospital security guard waited by the wall module to input the code for us — my guess is that the ER staff told him they had an impending delivery coming soon.

Bringing the pregnant woman out safely but swiftly, Ashley and I busted a gut towards the ER doors with the fireman stabilizing one side of the stretcher.

Just beyond the sliding ER doors, a physician stood at a time punching module — he was in the midst of clocking out. Recognizing our predicament, the ER physician turned his focus towards lending us a hand. "You guys must be headed to the L&D department (labor and delivery); I'll help you out before I go home, may as well." Fortunately, he happened to be in our line of travel and wanted to help; he possessed a security clearance card that we needed in order to even make it up to the floor labor and delivery was located on. Finding someone immediately available to escort us up to that floor could very well have been time-consuming — we were fortunate things happened the way they did with the physician.

"Hello, I'm Dr. Stevens… try to hold in any urges to push that baby out." Maria, in optimal distress, looked at Dr. Stevens as if he was out of his mind. "It will only take another two minutes or so to get to where we're going," the Doc reassured. Now entering an elevator, Maria repositioned herself. Opening her legs far and wide, she began to push. Dr. Stevens instantly put both of his hands on Maria's knees and closed her legs. "What is he doing??" I thought. I was a hair away from making a scene but decided to trust his judgment. Dr. Stevens' demeanor changed from easy-going to firm and rigid. "Listen to me," his voice lowered, "You are not having this baby inside this elevator… we are one minute away from the labor and delivery department." Maria became quiet; her eyes widened with fear. It was a bit unnerving to hear him be so stern with a pregnant patient getting ready to deliver. But at the same time, I'm positive Dr. Stevens has seen quite a few deliveries in his day — he was no novice, by any means.

The elevator doors opened, the double doors only 10 feet away was the labor and delivery entrance. Dr. Stevens swiped his card, prompting the double doors to electronically swing open. A nursing desk appeared with a nurse behind it, holding her arm out with a pointed finger. "That way, room number four," she directed. "Room number four…room number four… where are you already," I thought to myself. I heard multiple voices coming from an open door a few doors down the hallway. It was room number four! There were about seven nurses fully gowned and ready for action. "Please don't touch that table," one nurse warned cautiously. What she pointed to was a table with medical equipment laid out that absolutely had to remain sterile in order to use — equipment such as a scalpel, bulb syringe, chord clamps, etc.

"AAAYYYYYEEEE!! AAAYYYYYEEEE!!!" Maria screamed. Maria screamed so loud that the entire hospital must have heard her. She continued to yell at the top of her lungs, spreading her legs wide simultaneously. I glanced down to assess her vaginal opening as we lined the stretcher up right next to the L&D hospital bed — I saw what looked like a head protruding out from her vagina! I placed my gloved hand just below the baby's head to facilitate its delivery. One or two seconds passed by before Maria let out a sensational cry. "AAAYYYYEEE!!!" Maria screamed in her spanish accent. Out came the newborn baby. I clamped the cord and used the scalpel to sever it. A nurse standing next to me snatched up the newborn boy using a fresh towel. She dried him off and suctioned the nose and mouth. Everything happened all in one moment. Maria basically sneezed out the newborn — it shot out like a cannon, opposed to my first delivery, where it took the young woman multiple pushes to completely deliver the child.

Not with Maria though, not one bit. This was her *fourth* delivery; she undoubtedly was a seasoned veteran. "Congratulations Maria!" I said with a big smile. It was a true sight to behold, nature is really something. Maria, breathing heavily, kept her eyes closed as she panted. I'm not sure if she even heard my congratulatory statement. "I've never been a part of something like this," the fireman turned to me and said. "PSSHHH, me neither," Ashley blurted. "This is my first assisted delivery too, I'm still trying to figure out what exactly just happened." "Well… I better get going, I've gotta get back to the station," the fireman concluded. Standing there with his bunker pants and overalls, he extended his hand for a farewell handshake. "Thanks for all your help," I thanked him. "No problem, brother, I'll see you out there," he replied before turning to walk out the door. Ashley and I took the time to clean up our bloody cot. Our ambulance looked like a hurricane had hit it on the inside; we sanitized everything for the next call. "What a rush!" Ashley said with fire in her eyes. "It just goes to show, you never know what kind of call will be next!" I said. I can tell you what's next for me at the moment— Food! Let's get out of here, I'm hungry!" Ashley cried.

But he giveth more grace. Wherefore he saith, God resisted the proud, but giveth grace unto the humble. **James 4:6**

#55

He's In There...I Know He's In There

Paramedic Pointer» *Fevers, defined as 100.4 degrees Fahrenheit, are signs of infection. Fevers aren't necessarily a bad thing; they are a coping mechanism of the human body.*

Eccentric people are everywhere — you come to realize that in this line of work. *Abdominal Pain* was the chief complaint relayed to Jeff and I via our ambulance dispatch speaker. There are a myriad of reasons behind abdominal pain, especially with females. Abdominal pain for a female could translate to a full-blown heart attack because females present symptoms differently. It could also mean complications with a pregnancy.

Our patient was a large black woman named Memika. She lived on the backside of a duplex. Her front porch awning dripped a slow brown liquid that stained my uniform shirt. That's one of the perks you don't hear much about, they don't advertise that when inviting you to serve as a medic. Every environment has all sorts of fluids, droplets, scum, sweat, poop and pee you may very well come into contact with. Luckily, we've got washing machines and dryers to wash our uniforms when we get splattered with a pesky pile of puke. Disregarding my brown stained uniform, I continued inside to evaluate our patient.

Curled up on the sofa, our black female patient laid on her side, holding her abdomen. "What's going on today, hun?" I asked. She looked up at me, yet remained silent. "Hey I'm Lorenzo and this is my partner Jeff, we are your paramedics for today… what's going on with you?" I questioned her again. "…Uhhh…yeah… something is just not right. I had to come home from work early, which is unusual for me. I work 14 hour days…my heart just doesn't feel right… it's racing," she whispered under her breath. Stepping in closer to feel her wrist for a pulse, there didn't seem to be any abnormalities. The rhythm of the pulse was normal; the strength of her pulse was normal. And the rate didn't turn out to be accelerated like she felt it was. "Hmmm", I thought to myself, "maybe I'm missing something." I placed her on the cardiac monitor to assess her pulse and cardiac wave appearance — still nothing out of the ordinary. Memika's eyes remained squinted — just barely opened enough to see the brown irises she had.

She stayed frozen in her horizontal position of comfort across her couch. "Memika, I'm going to need you to get up and sit down on my stretcher, okay?" "My stomach hurts too bad…" she replied in a calm, effortless voice. Choosing to dig a bit deeper while still in the house, I asked, "What do *you* think the problem is today, Memika?" Did you maybe catch food poisoning? Did you ingest a new medication you've never taken before?" I attempted to draw out some clues. "I'm pregnant," Memika said subtly. "You're pregnant?" Jeff chimed in with curiosity. We both wondered why she wouldn't have said that in the first place. "Yes I'm pregnant." Jeff and I exchanged baffled looks with one another. "Uhh…how long have you been pregnant?" Jeff questioned. "For quite a few weeks now," she answered. "Have you taken one of those urine sample tests?" "… No." "Have you gotten an ultrasound done to show that you're pregnant??" Jeff asked with increased suspicion. "No," Memika replied. "Well then why do you feel that you're pregnant? What leads you to believe this?" he asked. "Because I can feel him inside." "You can feel him inside of you?" "Yesss…I can feel him in there kicking from time to time… he's in there…I know he is," Memika exclaimed. Jeff and I shot looks at one another for a second time, both of us sort of weirded out by the responses we were getting from this lady.

"How old are you, miss?" I asked, having pondered how old she was in my head for the past few minutes. "I'm 34. I was just discharged from the hospital about an hour ago. They checked me out and told me nothing was wrong. But I still feel terrible." "Wait a minute," I began, "You were just released from the hospital one hour ago and you want to go right back?" "Yes, because I still don't feel right. They didn't do anything for me," Memika said as she held up her ER wristband as proof that she had been seen. "They probably didn't do anything for you once they realized you were off your rocker," I thought. "Okay, if that's what you would like then that's what we'll do. We're here for you," I stated. None of Memika's vital signs were out of normal range. Her skin temperature was normal as well. Nothing appeared to be wrong. But something was certainly not adding up.

The typical person doesn't avoid a pregnancy test and instead go off of *their own* say-so. Even to be unaware of being pregnant until the baby is kicking is farfetched! It was a noneventful ride to the ER in the back of the truck, I basically monitored vital signs and that's about it. But get this, once we arrived at the hospital, nurses were giving the look of "not this woman again!" I explained everything to her receiving nurse — or at least I tried to — when the nurse interrupted me in midsentence. "Yes we saw her not too long ago. We deemed her to be a loose screw and sent her on her merry way." "Did you all do an ultrasound?" I said with a slight smirk. Rolling her eyes, she said, "No we didn't, but we will now just to check, since she's back again." Jeff and I had to prepare for our next call, so we had to run. When we came back with our next patient I asked the same nurse whether or not Memika was indeed pregnant or not. The nurse's reply was a slow, shameful head nod…NO.

The fear of the Lord is the instruction of wisdom; and before honor is humility. **Proverbs 15:33**

#56

Strange, Unsanitary Cyclops

Paramedic Pointer» *Do not use eye drops such as Clear Eyes to relieve irritated eyes. These eye drops constrict the blood vessels in your eyes, temporarily relieving redness, but end up making the issue worse. Use eye drops classified as "artificial tears", you can find these in the drug stores just as easily.*

Receiving a call marked as a *sick person* is like receiving study notes for a test, but when you look down, it's only a blank sheet of paper. In other words, there's no true way to prepare for calls that leave the nature of the call that vague on the computer screen in my ambulance. Yeah, sure, you got all your built-in knowledge as a paramedic you can draw from when you get there, but you can forget about knowing exactly what to expect before you arrive.

A full moon lit up the Florida sky at approximately 1:45 AM. I had only been in my station bed for 30 minutes or so when the alarm went off. Many of us don't enjoy being awoken out of our sleep, but in the world of EMS (emergency medical systems), one can expect to be woken up multiple times passed midnight. Just imagine someone saying, "Hey…hey it's time to wake up again" while shaking you — imagine this happening 2-5 times after midnight and you'll have an idea of how we paramedics are presented with emergencies throughout the nighttime hours. I never was the biggest fan of calls after midnight, and many other medics will tell you the same. After running a boat load of calls during the day, you'd like to be able to place your body's batteries on the charger (bed) to revamp. Fortunately it doesn't bother me *that* much at the end of the day; the job itself is a lot of fun.

The place I'm getting ready to tell you about sent chills down my spine, something about that moon when it's full brings out some real characters. What had to be one of the oldest apartment buildings in the entire county is where Jeff and I responded to this night. Extremely tall in stature, there was something like 25 floors when we looked at the operator panel from inside the elevator. Our patient was located on floor 19. Generally, the whole building was run down. Lights flickered, struggling to stay lit. Walls were old looking and torn in many spots throughout the structure. The integrity of the establishment was downright poor. I was waiting for it to come tumbling down into one big heap of rubble at any given moment. In fact, Jeff and I initially thought we were at the wrong place because the place looked abandoned!

Pressing the old elevator button, Jeff and I stood in silence as we rose to floor 19. –BING– The aged elevator chimed. It took forever and a day for those raggedy elevator doors to spread all the way open. Stepping out into the ridiculously long corridor, both Jeff and I took a brief moment to calibrate our eyes to the new lighting conditions. From one end to the next, the corridor we stood in (which seemed to be a mile long) was poorly lit. Every fourth ceiling light managed to remain lit up — but just barely. All other lights in between were completely off. "Does this place look abandoned or what?" I said to Jeff. "That ain't no joke," he replied.

Peering down towards the right end of the corridor we observed the door numbers to see which way counted upwards and vice versa. Peering back towards the left end of the mile-long corridor, we saw that based on how the other door numbers flowed, going left was our path to travel. Looking down that way as we began treading softly down the ghastly hallway, I noticed a figure. It was a dark figure, appearing to only be a shadow, due to the poor lighting. Honing in on the shadow figure, I made out a chair of some sort that the figure was sitting in.

Advancing further down the hall slowly revealed that it was a person in a wheelchair, rolling back and forth gently in the same spot. The person's position happened to be directly under one of the working ceiling lights — one of many that flickered in a struggle to stay on. In and out of the light, the person rolled, facing away from us, as we came down the spooky corridor wheeling our cot. By now I could tell that our *dark figure* was a man. Gently, he continued to roll back and forth, in and out of the light slowly. His movement and rhythm were robotic, the motion was so precise. Finally we made it all the way to the man. I was a bit nervous to walk around to the front side of the mysterious man's wheelchair — the whole scenario reminded me too much of a horror movie where something terrifying happens when the main character ventures off to investigate.

From his backside, I could already see that he didn't have a shirt on and the fact that he only had three stringy hairs sprouting from his bald head. What I saw next was unsightly to say the least, especially under the poorly lit conditions at 1:45 AM. A frozen, ear to ear grin, took up half of the man's face. His left eye was *missing* and he was completely naked. Hair engulfed the man's body from his shoulders down to his feet. "What's that smell?" Jeff candidly questioned aloud. "Wait — what is this stuff all over him?" Jeff continued. "It's feces," I told him, trying earnestly to hold my breath. The man's smile remained frozen, appearing to be plastered on his face. And I tell you no lie, he began giggling ever so softly as he continued to roll back and forth in his old wheelchair. He emulated the same rhythmic motion a rocking chair displays. "That is rank!" Jeff said, holding his nose. "Is there a yellow sheet on the back of the stretcher we can use to wrap this guy up in??" Jeff asked me. Our yellow sheets were specifically for predicaments such as this one. They subdued any salivation, lacrimation, urination, defecation, gastrointestinal contents, emesis or any other highly volatile bodily fluids.

There was no magic recipe or cleaning ingredients in our yellow sheets either. I'm talking about literally just wrapping a patient up like a burrito in their own filth so that the disdainful smell would stay at bay. "Yes, I see two yellow sheets back here we can use," I said leaning over to take a peek. Jeff and I spread it over our stretcher so that once we placed our patient on it, we could conveniently fold over the dangling ends. "Heehee-heehee-heehee," the old one-eyed man giggled as if he didn't have good sense. "What's your name sir?"

I asked. "…Heehee-heehee-heehee…" his skin temperature felt ice cold. "Can you hear me? I'd like to know what your name is and what's wrong today." "…Heehee-heehee-heehee" the bald man continued to giggle with his head thrown back. He appeared to be focusing on something on the ceiling but he wasn't — just an immovable, fixated gaze. At any moment, I anticipated him to latch onto one of us and try something absurd like bite a finger off.

"Who even called 911 for this strange man anyway?" I thought, as we wheeled him down the dark corridor. My guess is a frightened neighbor who heard his psychotic giggles outside of their door. They probably peeked through their peep hole and immediately dialed without opening their door. As far as any real medical concerns, outside of general infection due to his hygiene, we found nothing definitively wrong with the man. I mean, we did kinda conclude that he didn't exactly have all of his marbles upstairs, but who are we to diagnose someone as insane or mentally retarded? No abnormalities jumped out at us once we secured him in the back of the ambulance. I ended up pinching myself a few times en route to the ER. I thought that I must have been dreaming, and that at any second, I was going to wake up to find myself still under my comforter in my station bed.

Witnessing such an unusual combination of creepiness, chronic lack of hygiene, and eccentric character left me feeling uneasy. Receiving personnel at the ER felt likewise based off of the looks our patient got from them; and not to mention, us as well. "How has your day been so far?" I asked Misty, the ER nurse. "It's been bland, but it just got interesting," she said with her eyes opening wide. "What's going on with this fella?" she inquired. "Not much at all from what I can gather…he's pretty stable, but I'm sure you all's bloodwork will help reveal anything further." "Did you get a name, any medical history, allergies, etc.?" "No, you hear that sinister giggle he's got going on?" Misty nodded her head slowly, displaying a look of being generally disturbed. "Yeah, that's the extent of what I was able to salvage." "Ah-ha…" Misty replied. "Okay, I'll take it from here; did you need me to sign?" "Absolutely," I confirmed, presenting my toughbook (laptop) with the stylus so that Misty could sign for receipt of the patient. "See you next time," she gave a farewell. "Yep, until next time," I replied.

The Lord is with you, while ye be with Him; and if ye seek Him, He will be found of you; but if ye forsake Him, He will forsake you. **2 Chronicles 15:2**

#57

A Screaming Save

Paramedic Pointer» The compression rate for CPR is 100/ min for adults (Push hard and fast in the center of the chest). The compression-ventilation ratio is 30:2 (30 compressions: 2 Ventilations)

Anna Maria Island is generally a quiet place, even more so during the nighttime hours. Tonight turned out to be a deviation from the status quo. Our call came in as a seizure, but also said further down the computer dispatch screen, that the patient did *not* have a pulse. These are one of those instances when a paramedic just has to disregard his or her notes to a certain extent. It is likely that whoever phoned 911 never witnessed a seizure in person. I've seen CNA's who thought a patient with known Parkinson's disease (regular shakes) was undergoing a seizure. But when you don't know, you don't know, as they say.

Jeff and I arrived on scene to find a man whose entire head resembled a blueberry (sign of severe oxygen deprivation). He was laying on the side of the road in the crevice that reroutes rainwater into the sewers. A middle-aged female straddled him in the midst of a diehard attempt to resuscitate the downed man. From the ambulance cab, I could see how red the woman straddling our patient's face was. She was actively giving it everything she had, beads of sweat trickled down her face as she performed rapid chest compressions. "Looks like we'll be gettin' dirty," Jeff said as we stopped a few feet away from the patient. With no time to waste, we raced over to take control of the scene.

"Thank you Miss, we'll take it from here," I advised her, my adrenaline now pumping. I knelt down to feel for a pulse — nothing. "He's in cardiac arrest for certain! No pulses present!" I announced loud enough for Jeff and the on scene firemen to hear me. While one fireman began CPR in place of the middle-aged woman, I slapped on the defibrillation pads. "CHARGING!" I yelled. "IS EVERYONE CLEAR?" I glanced around to make sure. Jeff and the three firemen all had their hands up as if a policeman told them to "freeze." ZZZTT! "SHOCK DELIVERED! CONTINUE CPR!" I shouted. This particular man had crap for veins; I attempted twice but was unsuccessful.

In our paramedic toolbox is a drill called the *EZ-IO*. This tool is literally like a power tool. It is battery operated and works just like a power drill, only it drills a needle into one's bone marrow to gain access into a patient's bloodstream. "Since you're taking care of that, I'll go ahead and get the patient intubated (a tube placed in one's airway)!" Jeff advised. —PUMP-PUMP-PUMP-PUMP-PUMP— "Are you ready to switch John?" a fireman asked the other fireman performing CPR. "Yes, I'd appreciate it!" John replied. Switching positions quickly, the new fireman performing CPR made it apparent that his arms were fresh. He pumped like no tomorrow. And in a sense, there would be no tomorrow for our patient if we weren't successful in our resuscitation attempt. "My IO is good!" I loudly confirmed. IO stands for *intraosseous* — the medical term used to express *in the bone*.

I secured my access point and administered the initial drug. "The first epinephrine is in!" Moments later I called for a pulse check as I prepared to send a wave of electricity through our patient for a second time. "CHARGING!" I advised everyone. "IS EVERYONE CLEAR?!..." "WE'RE CLEAR", they each responded with their hands up. An important thing to note is that as professionals, safety comes first — on any level. Personal safety is paramount in the field. For instance, we paramedics always double, and sometimes triple check, that no one is in contact with the patient when the defibrillation (shock) is delivered. If someone mistakenly maintains contact when a defibrillation happens, they are in for a shock themselves! Surveying everyone once again to make sure there wasn't contact with our downed caucasian man, I pressed the button on my monitor....—SHOCK— The man's body jolted all at once — his arms and legs flew up in the air simultaneously and fell back down to the concrete.

"Continue compressions!" I directed. "Grab the backboard Jeff!" In order to properly move the man, we needed to place him on a rigid backboard. Rolling the patient to his left side, a fireman shoved the backboard under his backside before we rolled him back to a flat lying position. "One-two-three-Lift!" Jeff said from the foot end of the long backboard. In moving the pulse-less man into our truck, our lighting conditions improved tremendously. We went from working under the minimal lighting the moon provided to a fully illuminated patient compartment — "my office" as I like to call it. "Second dose of drugs given!" I told everyone. Allowing CPR to continue for two more minutes, I commanded a pause for a pulse check. "I've got a pulse!" I said with great surprise. Everyone lightened up just a hair. Hearing those words always offers relief to healthcare providers, it's what we long to hear. Like that three-point swish a basketball player dreams of making just before the game-ending buzzer concludes the game, we get a rush when someone is successfully resuscitated.

"Let's print out a picture of his heart please," I requested. The EKG (picture of the heart) began to print shortly after Jeff pressed the print button on our monitor. He began to give me what he found on the printout, when suddenly our patient's eyes opened and looked around. Our patient looked both confused and out of his mind. He gripped his airway tube (endotracheal tube) and attempted to pull it out. There is a bubble, or cuff, that we inflate to keep it locked into place, once we paramedics place it in a person's airway. I pried his hands open from the death grip he had on the tube and used my free hand to deflate the cuff I just mentioned. With an inflated cuff, a person could rip their throat out! Immediately after relieving the pressure from the cuff, I pulled the tube out of his mouth. "WOOOOH!....AAAHHHHH!....WOOOH....AAAAAHHHHHH!" the patient screamed. He screamed in a high-pitched tone that would make someone not looking at him believe he was a female. I've never seen a patient come back to a completely alert state after being revived. "Are you with us sir?" I asked, asking a rhetorical question to elicit a response other than his wailing. "AAAAHHHH!...WOOOOHH!... AAAHHHH...!!" The patient screamed with all his might. The screams reminded me of how someone would scream if they were on fire. The man had come back from the dead. There's no telling what he might have seen! Though he was highly audible, our patient was at a loss for *words*. All he could do the entire time was fill the air with those high-pitched screams.

He flailed all over the place on the way to the hospital, arms swinging around and around like windmills. The patient was nothing short of freaked out. —KSSHHHHH— the sound of air being released from the ambulance slowly hissed out as the back end lowered down; we were now at the ER. "WOOOHH! AAAHHHH! WOOOOH! AAAAAAHHHH!" our patient continued to cry. Finally making it into the ER room, Dr. Whorton came in, he was a dwarf-like man.

"Oh my, how long has he been carrying on like this, since you got a pulse back? I heard over the radio that you all were successful in resuscitating him, great job," Dr. Whorton commended us. Feeling for a pulse at the femoral artery (groin area), Dr. Whorton remarked, "Yep, we've got a strong pulse alright! This is a first; I've never seen someone this alive so soon after regaining a pulse... but I love it!" he concluded. It was indeed a unique outcome. Many survivors of cardiac arrest wind up living in a vegetative state. We turned over the care of our patient to the ER staff after moving the gentleman over to their bed. As I handed my toughbook (laptop) over to a nurse to sign for receipt of our patient, she commented, "You guys brought us a screamer!" Laughing, I turned to her and said, "You got that right... a screaming save!"

*The hand of our God is upon all them for good that seek Him; but His power and His wrath is against all them that forsake Him. **Ezra 8:22***

#58

A Hard Pill To Swallow

__Paramedic Pointer__» If a person is talking to you (or baby is crying), it is an optimal indicator that their airway is clear. One cannot choke and talk at the same time due to airway blockage.

We've heard the common phrase a person uses to explain why they are choking on their food: "I swallowed down the wrong pipe." But what does it *really* mean? In case it's never been spelled out for you, I'd like to clear the air briefly. There actually is a wrong pipe a person can swallow down. In the human throat there are two major pipes: one is your esophagus, which leads down to the stomach and the other pipe is your trachea — also known as the *windpipe*, which leads down to your lungs. Knowing this, you'd probably figure that the wrong pipe is the one leading down to the lungs (trachea). The trachea is that pipe people refer to in saying the "wrong pipe." When liquid or food slips into the trachea, aspiration tends to occur. This can happen when someone is asleep, not paying attention or just has poor motor control in regards to swallowing. Now that we've cleared up the air on that old saying, I'll tell you about a granny who mistakenly swallowed a pill that wound up getting lodged in the wrong place.

At 3 AM on a Tuesday night, Jeff and I awoke out of our sleep to rescue an older woman from none other than herself. Deciding to comply with her prescription pills regimen at such a late hour, she came across some difficulties. The neighborhood we responded to was an average, middle-class neighborhood. From the second we entered the patient's residence, I knew for sure it was an elderly person. In every room there were antique couches, the kind you never really sit on. "Back here!" an older gentleman's voice rang out from the back room. "Back here!" he yelled out again. Jeff and I followed the voice to find an old black couple lying in bed. In front of their king-sized bed sat a 65-inch television on a nightstand; they had the news on. Grandpa pointed to his wife and laid there in silence as if to say, "My job's done, I can relax now."

Granny sat up as soon as we passed through the doorway into her bedroomroom. "Mm-mmmm….mm-mmmmm!" she moaned. "What's in your mouth, dear?" I asked. Clearing his throat, grandpa sat up to rest on his elbows and said, "She swallowed a pill down the wrong pipe… I told her everything would be fine, but she insisted on calling you guys… I said, well, I'd better leave it alone if she's that serious about getting help!" grandpa eased back down to lay flat on his back. "Open your mouth and stick out your tongue for me Miss," I prompted our female patient. "AHHHHH…" Grandma hung her tongue down while I took a look inside her mouth with a penlight. Nothing came into view but the external drool running down the corner of grandma's mouth. "Can you feel what area the pill is in in your mouth?" I questioned. "Mm-mmmm….mm-mmmmm!" Grandma moaned while pointing towards the back of her throat.

Her indiscernible moans sounded like she was trying to say, "Right here!" Right about now is when a change of mood occurred out of nowhere. Jeff was typing in information on the laptop when a 4 foot body grazed across his pant leg. "Oh…hey…!" Jeff said, initially startled out of his skin. A black child, who had to be no more than 9 or 10, speed walked into his grandparents' room with two bawled up fists. His head was tilted downward slightly — he had his angry face on! The young boy's face was scrunched up so much that his eyebrows almost touched in the middle. "What's going on with this fella?" I thought to myself. He looked like he was one second away from swinging on Jeff. And then something out of left field occurred — suddenly the boy's angered facial expression faded into one of compassion. He inched closer and closer to Jeff's leg with his *Batman* bed slippers on and gave Jeff a long, drawn out hug of affection.

"Is this kid sleepwalking or is he just nuts?!" I thought. The young boy then scooted along to the far corner of his grandparents' bed and hopped in. "What are you doing up at this hour Terrell?" his grandfather said with a smirk on his face. Turning the focus completely back onto granny, I leaned down to take one more look with my penlight. "I don't see anything Miss, it's too far down apparently." She shook her head in a bit of frustration and grew silent, waiting for me to serve her the conclusion of the matter. "I know how concerned you are dear, but I've got good news… you're going to be just fine — you'll just have to wait until that pill dissolves." Grandma wore two hearing aids. "Does she normally speak well?" I asked her husband. Shaking his head vigorously, he said no. "She's hard of hearing and it's so bad that when she speaks, she doesn't actually say words." "That makes sense," I thought.

The pill was not altering her ability to talk; making garbled noises was normal for her. "Take a deep breath through your mouth, hun," I instructed her. Her inhale and exhale sounded free and clear, confirming that her airway was not blocked. "Your airway isn't blocked, Miss, that was my primary concern. With that being said, your vital signs are fantastic and you won't need to go to the hospital unless you want to." Giving herself a moment to ponder the decision, she shook her head from side to side and moaned, "Mm-mmm" as if to say "uh-uh" or "no". "If you need us to come back, remember, we're here for you… call us back if you need us at any time and we'll come right back out!" Grandma signed the refusal document on my touchscreen laptop once she decided on staying home.

On our way out, Jeff began to chuckle. "What's up?" I inquired. "Man! I thought I was going to get punched in the face by a 10-year-old!" "It probably would have been good for you… it would have woke you up all the way," I said, noticing that Jeff had crust in the wears of his eyes still. "Good thing too, because I can't fight, what would my wife think if I went home and told her I got beat up by a kid??" "Those kinds of things you seal tightly in a box and bury them," I said with laughter. "You just take those types of embarrassments to the grave."

But if from thence thou shalt seek the Lord thy God, thou shalt find Him, if thou seek Him with all thy heart and with all thy soul. **Deuteronomy 4:29**

#59

Superhuman Strength

Paramedic Pointer» *The gag reflex protects fluids or solids from going into the lungs. The eyelash reflex is a fairly reliable indicator of the presence or absence of an intact gag reflex. If the patient's lower eyelid contracts when you gently stroke the upper eyelashes, he or she probably has an intact gag reflex.*

Anytime drugs are involved with the patient, things have a propensity to become elevated. The waters that were originally clear and calm can quickly transform into murky waters. Lines get blurred. Things become obscure and fuzzy. We've all heard of the carelessness people convey while on drugs — and the consequences they incur from acting on those irrational impulses. One instance many were disturbed by was the man down in the Miami, Florida area who had infamously earned the name *zombie*. This gentleman decided to eat away a man's face while he was high on bath salts. Pretty gross right? Drugs or no drugs, you've got to be one mentally disturbed individual to go through with that kind of obscene behavior.

There's a whole host of drugs one can get into: there's *prescription drugs, over-the-counter drugs, recreational drugs, compliance drugs, herbal drugs, exercise supplemental drugs* and much more! You got your *hypnotics, sedatives, anesthetics, psychedelics, hallucinogens, antidepressants, uppers, downers,* you name it.

Me and my on scene posse couldn't quite put a finger on exactly what this particular man was on, but we did know that it gave him extraterrestrial strength to resist our advances of medical care. He was located in an alleyway that was very close to pitch black. We were notified that there was a man sitting in a vehicle, blocking through- traffic next to an apartment complex. Apparently someone needed to pass through but was playing it safe because my dispatch notes read, "Caller states they will not get close to vehicle in dark alley."

Jeff and I turned on to the designated block the call was located on. We scanned the block slowly, peering down each alleyway with squinted eyes to spot our said vehicle. Slowly rolling passed the third dark alleyway on the block, there it was — a red pickup truck with the headlights dimmed. The two streets perpendicular to the alley were lined with streetlights but the alley itself had none. All there was was the silent darkness of the alleyway with a lone red truck parked in the center. On the corner of the apartment complex, a young woman and an older gentleman stood, talking vigorously to one another. Their body language looked as if they were discussing the mysterious red truck in the alley next to their complex. I saw the young woman, who was wearing blue jeans and a gray sweater, quickly turn around to glance at the red pickup truck and continue her conversation with the older gentleman.

As we turned into the alley, they both looked up as if they had just become aware of Jeff and I in the humongous ambulance — as if they had not heard or seen our truck easing down the block from the beginning. The woman in the gray sweater motioned us to roll down our window. Pressing the button to make the passenger window retract into the door, the woman approached my side saying, "Over there…" she pointed. "There's a really strange man with music on sitting in his car… he's looking straightforward, bobbing his head back and forth." "How long has he been there, do you know?" "I'm not sure, I go into work at midnight; I work the graveyard shift. I just noticed him when I was pulling out to leave for work… normally I use the alley to snake through to the next street over, but not tonight… I'm not sure what that guy has going on!" she exclaimed. "Not a problem, we'll go and check things out," I assured her.

We parked the ambulance a few yards away from the mysterious man and dismounted our truck. "It's a full moon out today," I thought. "Please don't let this be a madman we have to deal with at this hour." Jeff and I kicked up dust as we walked towards the red truck to see what was up. The head-bobbing the young woman described had just ceased. He sat there now, appearing to be expended of all his vital energy. Peering into his window to identify any weapons he might have, Jeff said, "He doesn't seem to be armed with anything so that's a start." I shined my flashlight onto the driver's door handle and stood just to the right of the door, leaning my hip onto the car. "He wet himself," Jeff proclaimed, when he stepped inside the now ajar door. In the passenger seat sat a small plastic baggie with white powder in it. I shined the flashlight all around the truck's cloth interior—first the front row and then the back seats. Up and down I shined the flashlight on our patient from head to toe.

There was snow white powder on his nose and the remainder of it made a small trail from his T-shirt's collar down to his belly. "It looks like he overdid it to me," I told Jeff. Coupling the urine drenched jeans and the head bobbing the young woman witnessed, it was a great possibility that the patient conjured up a seizure while playing in the cocaine. Jeff and I lifted the patient out of his vehicle and laid him on our cot. He still had a pulse and was actively breathing, even though he was unresponsive. Dust flew up from that old dirt road as we made our way towards our ambulance. Had you been trailing behind us you'd have seen every particle of dust with perfect clarity thanks to the bright headlights from the ambo that nearly blinded us both. "This guy really outdid himself tonight… something about those full moons I tell ya," Jeff stated. The rocky gravel and dirt made for a rough trek from the gentleman's truck to the rear of the ambo.

Our patient flinched as we loaded him into the back. It appeared as if he was waking up, but he never opened his eyes. He sort of snatched his forearm towards his chest as if to prepare a backhand swing on somebody. Right then and there Jeff and I both sensed a violent aura coming from him. I could tell Jeff felt exactly how I did because the look he gave me was the same look I gave him — a look of thankfulness that the man didn't wake up. Apparently our fire engine responding to this call got lost because they were just now arriving to the scene. "Sorry we're late guys!" one of the three firemen in overalls apologized candidly. "We were given the wrong address!" He continued. Normally by the time a patient was placed in the back of the ambulance we would cut the firemen loose because they didn't do any transporting to hospitals, only we did.

Special cases would warrant a fireman (or two) to ride along with us to the hospital, namely calls where extra hands were a necessity. Standing outside the ambulance rear doors, one of the three firemen said, "Do you want any help?" Considering the eerie vibe I got from this patient, it didn't take much thought before I responded adamantly. "Yeah, you guys better stick around just in case; I got a funny feeling about this one." "You got it chief," he replied, hopping into the back of the rig. Everyone gathered vital signs while I obtained IV access. The moment after I sealed off his IV and taped it down, the anonymous man began thrashing all over the place. "Let me go! Let me go!" he yelled in a madman's tone. He gazed at me with the stare of a psychopath, displacing his bottom jaw forward exposing his bottom row of teeth — much like that of an alpha male wolf or lion that wants his prey to be sure that they have sharp teeth to do real damage with.

I was so happy that he had remained unconscious through the IV process — all of the violent flailing he was doing now could have caused me to poke myself with my own needle. Jeff and the three firemen jumped on each of the man's extremities, though it took everything they had just to hold down one limb. "Grab the restraints Lorenzo!" Jeff desperately cried. Five or six packages fell out of the restraints cabinet as I opened it — there was a surplus of limb restraints just waiting to be used — they had accumulated little by little over time from crews ordering them, but rarely using them. In one motion I bent down to scoop the packages up and began to tear them open. "His legs are super strong!" One fireman grimaced with his forehead vein protruding. "So is his arms; what did you take?!" another fireman asked while straining to keep his limb down.

The wild patient was in no mental state to answer any questions, nor cooperate in any way. "Hurry Lorenzo!" the nearest fireman urged me. I slapped on the restraint and tied a firm knot. I repeated this three more times — one restraint per limb as the patient cussed, yelled and threatened to kill us all if we didn't let him go. Once all of his extremities were secured, the man thrusted his head and chest forward with all of his might. "LET ME GO! LET ME GO!" he continually screamed as if we were miles away from him. His thrashing continued for about three minutes or so, I was impressed with his persistence — especially since he likely had a seizure. Most seizure patients are as weak as they can possibly be in the post-seizure stage. The tenacious thrashing about pointed towards his little white baggie of joy he had sitting in his passenger seat.

I drew up a vial of *Haldol* — a drug that would calm him down. No later than when the last droplet of the medication entered my syringe did I wait to poke him in his shoulder and shove the dosage of Haldol into him. The wild man continued to jolt and jerk. We all monitored him closely with our faces dripping with sweat. One fireman, whose sweat dripped copiously from his beak of a nose, stood there with both hands on his hips in awe. You could tell that he was drained. "How long does that Haldol take to kick in?!" the drained fireman asked. Silence overcame the patient right at that moment. The patient attempted to fight the sedative effects, but did not prevail. Instead, he slowly faded into a serene slumber. "Two of you should ride with us just in case; the Haldol is supposed to work for a decent amount of time but just to be on the safe side, come along. Something tells me this guy is strong enough to bust through those restraints if he wakes up again!" We crept carefully down the city streets to the ER—hoping against hope—that our dragon of a patient did not return to a fully alert state.

Blessed is he that readeth, and they that hear the words of this prophecy, and keep those things which are written therein: for the time is at hand. **Revelation 1:3**

#60

Skate Park Competitions

***Paramedic Pointer*»** *Children younger than 3 years of age incur fewer injuries from falls greater than three stories than do older children and adults, most likely because of the more elastic nature of their tissues and less ossification (bone formation). They are much like gummy bears, tending to bounce rather than break.*

"What a sunny day out, eh?" Jeff admired the clear blue skies from the driver seat of the ambulance on a Saturday afternoon. We were on a standby at a much anticipated skating competition held at a local skate park in zone 16. This particular skate park had to be a skater's dream. It was located right on the water; the view was a real beauty. Right next to the fashionable skate park was a sanded area with volleyball courts. The park itself seemed to have been built for recreational competition, and indeed it was competition in style. Palm trees surrounded the entire park on both the volleyball side and the skate park portion. Elegant canopies placed throughout the properties provided optimal shade for the park's visitors. Landscaping, in general, was exceptionally impressive, one could tell that a lot of money went into beautification and upkeep of the public property.

One by one, we watched skateboarders launch themselves into the air from a half pipe ramp. So many flips, twists and 360s were done that it left both Jeff

216

and I's bottom jaw on the floor. "You know, I never understood the interest in hopping on a skateboard and flying up and down tall ramps. How do you even practice that without getting injured?" I said with a light chuckle. "I busted my butt pretty bad on a pair of skis back in Chicago when I lived there… that was it for me!" Jeff said as he shook his head. "Nope… never was much of the athletic type," Jeff added. "It's probably why this has only gotten bigger and bigger with time," Jeff said as he rubbed his gut. Jeff wasn't lying about his lack of athletic ability, you could even tell from the way he walked. His gait was clumsy, far from anything someone with coordination would walk like. He wasn't obese, but at the same time, Jeff didn't involve himself in much physical activity outside of the exercise he received from running 911 calls every third day.

"Up, there goes another one," Jeff pointed out of the driver-side window. It's only a matter of time before one of them wipe out. As nonchalant as Jeff made the statement — he was right. I've seen it all before. What I've concluded from all my experience in EMS is this: *where many people gather, accidents will occur*. It's inevitable. Football games, concerts, competitions, church, etc., something emergency related is bound to occur. "If we're going to be cooped up in this box for the duration of this event, we may as well enjoy the fresh air," Jeff concluded. We both rolled our windows all the way down and took in the refreshing breeze. Just moments later we heard a loud thud followed by an audible *crunch*. "Yep, that sounds like a fracture," Jeff said. At the bottom of the ramp inside the half pipe laid a young blonde male with a bandanna on his head. He was holding his leg with squinted eyes as he bit down viciously on his bottom lip. Jeff and I jumped out of the ambulance so fast that I nearly tripped down from almost missing the step that helps you dismount the rig safely. Multiple skaters fled to the young blonde boy who fought to hold back his tears. "Are you okay bro… yeah, are you okay man?" are what the whispers from the crowd translated to. "Everyone backup!" I shouted as we approached the downed skater. "Where are you hurting?" I asked our patient. "… It's my ankle… this one…" he pointed to his left foot while straining to keep his composure. His injured ankle was swollen and purple colored.

In comparison to his right ankle, his left ankle was easily twice the size. "Did you feel a snap or a crunch?" "Yes, it feels like my ankle is broken…" he said painfully. "Grab a pillow for him, will you Jeff?" I said. "We'll place your ankle on a pillow until we get you inside our truck to give you some meds," I told the skater. The patient's blonde hair covered his ears entirely, draping over his shoulders and beyond. "Is it broken?" he asked me. "We don't have an x-ray machine to confirm fractured bones, but I can tell you that I'm about 99.9% sure that your ankle is fractured. What would you say your pain is right now on a scale of 1 to 10, 10 being the worst pain you've ever felt in your entire life?"

By now the adolescent boy had gathered much more composure and propped himself up on his elbows, "Uhh, I'd say about a 6 out of 10; I think I'm going to be able to handle it just fine dude," he said with a now faint smile. I'm aware that it's more macho to downplay pain when in the presence of your buddies, so I assumed that this was the stance our patient was trying to take. "What's your name by the way buddy?" "Tyler," he answered. "As a matter of fact, is there any way I can go to the hospital by having my mom take me? I don't need any pain meds or anything do I?"

"That depends on whether you feel you need them or not... they are certainly an available option to you with your mechanism of injury," I stated. "Thanks, but I think I'll be just fine without them dude," Tyler said with a geeky smile on his face that reflected a high level of confidence in his decision. "This kid is actually serious," I thought to myself, once we relocated to the back of my rig. What I thought to be a macho man *front* turned out to be no front at all! Tyler was genuinely prepared to manage the pain all by himself. Tyler, Jeff and myself waited patiently for Tyler's mom to arrive, with Tyler only being 17 (a minor), he wasn't old enough to sign a refusal of transport.

Balancing on one leg with one arm around his mother when she arrived, Tyler hopped along to get in his mother's car. "Thanks bro," Tyler thanked us before getting ready to sit down in the vehicle. "Do you want to keep your icepack macho man?" I questioned. That was the only intervention we took while waiting for Tyler's mother to arrive. "Sure, toss it over," he replied, his head just far enough above the passenger door to be visible. "Here you are macho man," I said, tossing the ice pack to him. "Be safe out there... from now on you're going to have to land those tricks; too many of these kinds of accidents will take you out your career!" Tyler looked at me and laughed.

For the word of God is quick, and powerful, and sharper than any two-edged sword, piercing even to the dividing asunder of soul and spirit, and of the joints and marrow, and is a discerner of the thoughts and intents of the heart. **Hebrews 4:12**

#61

Beaten With A Bat

Paramedic Pointer» *Ligaments connect bone to bone; tendons connect muscle to bone.*

Of all the cruel and unusual punishments a person can dream up, using a baseball bat to assault someone has got to be ranked pretty high. My guess is that someone has to piss another person off pretty darn bad to drive an individual to swing on them with a *Louisville slugger*. With men, money and infidelity are two big reasons their anger could reach its boiling point.

I once talked to two paramedics in one week about infidelity. These two gentlemen were much older; they both had been in a 20 year marriage. Coincidentally, their marriages ended the exact same way. In both instances, they had let an old friend who was down and out, stay at their houses for a couple of months. Lo and behold, time revealed that their old best friends were having relations with the wife. One of the paramedics said his wife broke the news to him on Christmas — she must have had a heart made of ice. The relations went on while the paramedics were at work. We paramedics work a 24/48 hour shift rotation. In other words, we work 24 hour shifts while on duty and get 48 hours off. It's a neat schedule because every time we work it's virtually the weekend again the following two days.

It's a shame infidelity has to happen; no one — man or woman — should have to put up with the unsettling thoughts of being cheated on while at their workplace. While were on this topic, I'd like to offer some advice on the matter: your best bet in marriage is to marry a God-fearing man or woman.

So it was approximately 1 AM when we received a call for an assault. Every single shift in zone 16 proved to be inescapable that an assault would occur. At some point after nightfall, some brawl or bashing happened without fail. Our dispatch notes revealed that a man had been brutally beaten with a bat and that there was bleeding involved — *large* amounts at that. There must've been 20 people or so at the scene when we arrived; it was almost like we were playing *Where's Waldo* on a smaller scale because the patient seemed to be nowhere in sight. There were an uncanny amount of people bunched up together. Jeff and I soon learned, however, that the amount of people was not what made locating our patient difficult. What made finding the victim difficult was that our patient was under a pickup truck resting facedown. The gentleman laid there with pure terror in his eyes, whimpering ever so audibly. I could tell that he was still on watch for his aggressor by the look in his eyes when I knelt down to take a look under the truck. Tension left his body when he realized that I was not his enemy, but a paramedic there to help him.

Even though it was dark out and he was up under a pickup truck, I could make out a small pool of blood under his left leg. Kneeling down beside me, Jeff said, "That left leg has a joint where a joint isn't supposed to be… look at his shin… can you see that?" he asked me. "Yes, I see it." Our patient's shin, instead of being straight as an arrow, was angled like a *triangle*. He suffered an open compound fracture from the person delivering blows with the baseball bat. Only a few times have I seen fear in someone's eyes to this degree. I was reluctant to pull him out from under the truck because I knew avoiding pain was out of the question. There was no possible way to start an IV on him to deliver morphine or dilaudid because of how he was positioned. I would have to literally crawl under the truck with a flashlight and attempt an IV with little room and lighting.

"What a disaster," I thought to myself. It's typically a standardized practice to induce pain medication before manipulating an injury such as this one. But it had to be done. If this man was going to receive any advanced medical treatment whatsoever, he would need to be accessible, which meant dragging him out into the open. "Are you ready to move him?" Jeff turned and asked me. He could tell my discomfort in the matter by my brief hesitation before grabbing a hold of the middle-aged man's belt loop. "Yeah, I'm ready when you are," I replied. My heart dropped the second we began to tug on our patient's body. I expected him to cry out in an agonizing cry of distress, but to my surprise, he merely moaned. And the moan wasn't a loud one. No, not at all. It was more like a soft moan of a little old lady who had non-traumatic back pain.

"This guy is either tough as nails or has completely lost sensation to his left leg," Jeff said. Moving his leg made me quiver ever so slightly, and I am by no means, one who is squeamish. It was such a freakish feeling to hold someone's leg and it collapse into two separate pieces instead of remaining intact. Now that we had him out from under the truck, I began preparing to start an IV in his arm when Jeff held me up with a small request. "Can you hold his leg stable for a moment?" He quickly asked me. "Sure," I replied as I firmly supported his fractured tibia (front shin bone) from the underside of his calve. The shin bone (tibia) was clearly visible outside of the patient's skin. It's one thing to know that bones exist inside the human body, but it's a whole new ballgame when they are poking out at you with sharp, bloodied marrow that could be used to stab someone.

Holding the injured man's calve, Jeff began to pull traction on the disconnected bones. Interestingly enough, it snapped right back into place! For a second time now, I expected to hear the falsetto cry of the century from our patient, but only a faint hum surfaced. Proceeding with the IV, the middle-aged Mexican male had many excellent veins to choose from. They were as thick as pipes; there was no chance of missing the stick. "Give me the morphine would you," I prompted Jeff. (I always find myself placing myself in the position of the patient to try and give myself the same sense of urgency I would appreciate if I were in their shoes). Doing this tends to keep me on a very fast pace when I'm working. In school, they tell you remember that it's not *your* emergency in order to maintain a level head.

Also, it's an effort to reduce work-related injuries such as poking yourself with a needle or rushing into an unsafe environment. We gave the patient a generous dose of morphine, followed by a generous dose of dilaudid. The goal was to make the patient snowed (very high) so that he was barely aware that he endured such a traumatic fracture. After wrapping the patient's shin with a leg splint, we made haste to load him into the rear of the ambulance. The only treatment left for this particular patient, for the most part, was active monitoring and the burning of diesel fuel as we sped to the ER. Jeff and I left the scene of 20 people — mostly women — bawling profusely. There were enough tears left behind at the scene to give the Atlantic Ocean a run for its money.

As newborn babes, desire the sincere milk of the word, that ye may grow thereby. **1 Peter 2:2**

#62

Pick Her Butt Up!

Paramedic Pointer» *Liquid drug forms include: solutions, suspensions, fluid extract, tinctures, spirits, syrups, elixirs, milk, emulsions, liniments and lotions.*

Not every call is a life-saving event. The reality of EMS is that there are a lot of responses that don't necessarily demand an ambulance. And unfortunately, just like not every call requires an ambulance, not every call is accompanied by polite people. You'd think that if an individual is asking for help, they'd at least have the decency to talk to the emergency responders with a certain level of respect. Apparently that's asking a bit too much for some people. One of the calls we paramedics find ourselves responding to here in the state of Florida is the issue of falls. There are trip and falls, slip and falls, roll out of bed falls, falls because people are obscenely obese and have no balance, and of course those psychiatric patients who *believe* they are falling. Let's not forget falls that occur simply from old age. Here in Florida, we are overly saturated with elderly people who come here to retire. I want to tell you about one elderly couple, in particular, because I was absolutely shocked at the behavior by one of them — namely the husband.

It was a sunny afternoon in the trailer park Jeff and I received a call from. Our notes advised that the female patient would only need a lift assist (help getting off the ground). The catch to this seemingly simple task was that she was 460 pounds. Her husband and she was an odd couple in my opinion, but then again, they say opposites attract. Let me put it to you this way: if the couple were standing next to one another, they would look like the number 10. The fire crew was dispatched to this call since we would need an extra couple pairs of hands in lifting the fallen woman back into her recliner as she requested. It might not have been so bad if she was actually *close* to her recliner. The way she asked about being put back into recliner would make one think it was nearby; but we were way on the opposite side of the house in a narrow hallway that she barely fit inside of!

Not a full minute had gone by when we entered the home before an angry grandpa in overalls, who resembled a skeleton in physique, stormed throughout the house with a snarly demeanor. Pacing vigorously throughout the home, he intermittently snatched his head upward to shoot us dirty looks. There were actually three paramedics: Jeff, myself and a new girl named Beth who was training with us. We all looked at each other with an expression that said, "What on earth is wrong with this guy?" The vibe inside the home was an uneasy one from the get-go. "Pick her up!" The husband shouted, wiping his runny nose shortly thereafter. The three of us stood still — appalled at the husband's unscrupulous behavior. "What are you all looking at?! Are you three gonna do your jobs or just stand there frozen in time?! Pick her up! Pick her up, you imbeciles!" the scrawny old man barked before storming around the corner with his hands on his hips.

Beth decided to give the old man a piece of her mind. "Excuse me Sir! You need to calm down! We're here to help your wife out and you are being extremely disrespectful! Now stop talking to us that way!" The patient's husband came speed walking from around the corner, hands still on his hips, and shouted, "Shut up and do your job you stupid idiot!" pointing his finger now with one hand still on his hip. He immediately turned away from her to storm back around the corner. "I'm going to my room now! You all deal with this before I send you guys back in exchange for another crew..." his voice faded as he got further away. "Let's go ahead and call to see where our fire crew is at before we try to do anything," I turned and told Jeff. Jeff took a brief moment to consult with our en route fire unit so that we knew when our extra pairs of hands would arrive. Their ETA (estimated time of arrival) was 3 to 5 minutes. Staring at our fallen female patient in the hallway was like seeing an extra-large hot dog that barely fit into its bun. She was lying face down with the two walls hugging her sides— it's no wonder she had been short of breath. "Do we have the patient mover on the back of the stretcher?" I asked, hoping to be proactive before the fire crew got there. "No, we trashed the last one, but there is a spare on the truck," Jeff answered. The patient mover is exactly what its name implies — it *moves* patients. The running joke, or alternate name, rather, in the private EMS world is the *whale mover* (or shampoo mover), referring to the morbidly obese patients. Jeff ran out and quickly returned with the patient mover in hand. I wanted to get our patient positioned onto the patient mover before the firemen arrived so that then all we'd have to do was muscle her over to her recliner.

Getting the mover underneath the obese patient was a real challenge. We stuffed and stuffed and stuffed some more. We ended up having to tilt her on her side to get it all the way under her good enough. By the time she was evenly centered on to our mover, the firemen arrived. It was a good thing too, because the three of us (Jeff, myself and Beth) were drenched in sweat. The aroma of our body odor coupled with the patient's body odor began to marinate, creating one big cloud of funk. "Where do you need us?" the first fireman entering the area said. "Now that there's six of us here, we can each grab one handle a piece and lift! But first, let's slide her out of this hallway so that we have more room to work with," I explained. It was almost like a tug-of-war battle trying to unplug her wide body out from the jaws of that corridor.

"NOOOO!" The woman let out a startling sound effect. She began breathing heavily — I thought she was going to have a panic attack. "Give her a moment guys," I cautioned. Now she lay on her back in the midst of the kitchen floor. Giving it a minute or two, we all regained our bearings for a dead lift. And not only was it a hefty lift, but we had to walk all the way to another room with her. "One, two, three…LIFT!" I urged everyone. Luckily, with six helpers, the carry wasn't all that bad. Our main difficulty came from our limited space due to the trailer home being so tight.

We placed her as far back into her recliner as we possibly could; we didn't want there to be any chance of sliding out of the chair, on to the floor. Her vital signs came back just fine and she didn't even wait until her evaluation was done before turning on the television. The patient's husband came out of his room now walking slowly with tears in his eyes. His steps were slow, stutter steps — like a three-year-old takes when they are unsure of themselves. Full of sorrow, I could see that he had shame in his heart. "Hey guys... look, I'm sorry for how I behaved a bit ago... it's just that I get so worried when my wife falls... I'm too old and weak to pick her up," he apologized. "And I'm so sorry for calling you out of your name... please forgive me," he said to Beth. Beth said, "no problem, I know how things can get in stressful times... thank you for your apology."

Our female patient's face brightened once she tuned in to her television program. As soon as she tuned in, she tuned all of us *out*. Going to the hospital was the last thing on her mind. And with no abnormal assessment findings, the ER had no justifiable reason to be on her mind. No transport necessary.

The holy Scriptures, which are able to make thee wise unto salvation through faith which is in Christ Jesus. All Scripture is given by inspiration of God, and is profitable for doctrine, for reproof, for correction, for instruction in righteousness.
2 Timothy 3:15 – 16

#63

Do You Feel Her Pain?

Paramedic Pointer» *Solid drug forms include: extract, powders, pills, capsules, pulvules, tablets, suppositories, ointments, and patches.*

I've been privileged to witness camaraderie on many a calls throughout my endeavors in the world of emergencies. Most of the time that camaraderie that I speak of is between husband and wife or girlfriend and boyfriend. Sometimes it's the pets of the patient that show that through the *thick and the thin* sort of bond. Too many times I've seen that final kiss goodbye, accompanied by those sacred words, "I love you." One single woman had a dog that refused to leave her side — through her medical evaluation and all — he was stuck to her hip the entire time she sat on her sofa.

But one patient showed no tolerance for her best friend (the patient) talking to us at all — even though her best friend was the one with the emergency. So as the story goes, we get a call for a possible broken hip. A woman by the name of Sidney took a fall and fractured her hip late one Sunday night. Scents of whiskey and vodka emitted from the pores of all of the visitors' skin — everyone was wasted. A group of friends had gotten together to get plastered with alcohol apparently, everyone reeked of liquor. A man standing in front of the kitchen bar held up a pointed finger — his other hand holding a beer — directing us to go to the room on the left. There lying in the bed was a middle-aged woman whose facial expression told us she was in severe pain. Another woman lay on her side, right next to the distressed patient. She intertwined her legs like a pretzel as she lay on her side with one hand gently resting on the patient's stomach.

"Hello, I'm Lorenzo and this is my partner Jeff… we'll be your paramedics for today. So what's going on with you Miss?" I asked the woman who was blatantly in discomfort. —"Oh, hello you guys, I'm her best friend Sarah, we go back years and years and years," she said with lazy eyes. She smiled as big as anyone could smile, but she couldn't hide how much she had to drink by her drunken sway and lazy eyes. "Sidney fell down the stairs when we were coming down them." "How many steps would you say she fell down?" I asked. "I don't know, maybe five or six…" Sarah said as she fought to maintain control of her heavy eyes.

Meanwhile, Sidney (the patient) kept quiet, choosing not to say anything at all to us. "I think she broke her hip because she can't get up at all…we had to carry her in here," Sarah said referring to the bedroom all of us were in. When hips get fractured, there's no downplaying that it's painful. But I can't say I've ever known a hip fracture to abade someone's ability to speak to my partner and me. I was still trying to figure out why her drunk best friend was doing all the talking for Sidney. Sidney didn't seem to be drunk at all — just in pain. We assessed Sidney's legs for something called *shortening*. Shortening is exactly how it sounds; a person's broken hip causes one leg to be shorter than the other. Sydney's left leg was definitely shorter than the right. I felt her pelvic region using both of my hands; one hand on each side of her hips, and I could feel the huge difference when comparing each side.

"Hand me our narcotic box, Jeff," I said. First things first — we had to get Sidney juiced up with some potent medication because a broken hip is not to be confused with something minor such as a stubbed toe or a scraped knee. "I'm going to start an IV in your arm and give you some drugs before we move you okay…? I can tell that your hip is broken…I mean, I'm not an x-ray machine by any measure, but I do know a broken hip when I see one". Sydney continued to lie flat on her back, in silence, making an occasional moan of discomfort.

Her best friend, Sarah, continued to tell of how long they had been good friends and how she would never turn her back on Sidney. And Sarah said something out of the ordinary — the funny part was that she thought she was being helpful. Sarah began running her fingertips along Sidney's thigh. My instant thought was, "What is this lady doing?" Sarah, with a serious look on her face, said, "Sidney's pain is all up and through here…can you feel her pain?"

—Okay wait a minute.

"Did this woman just say what I think she said?" I thought to myself. Jeff and I exchanged looks with one another. "What…?" Jeff questioned the best friend lying next to Sydney. "Her pain is up and through here… can you feel that pain?" Sarah repeated herself, maintaining a dead serious demeanor. Realizing that the woman was clearly speaking drunken nonsense, Jeff decided to play along and agree with her question. "Eeeeyeeeah…" he replied. "Look, I'm going to need you to move so that I can start this IV and get her onto my cot," Jeff said, speaking to Sarah. "Oh absolutely," she replied.

Our pain meds now on board (in the patient's body), we used the flat sheet Sidney was laying on to ease her over to our stretcher. It wasn't a bad transition at all. We lined up the cot next to the queen size bed so that there was no gap and slid Sidney on over. Even up until we got out to the truck, the best friend Sarah was talking our ears off about irrelevant jibber jabber. She digressed from talking about the patient to talking about herself. Alcohol tends to mix things up, that's for sure. But at the end of the day, she didn't interfere with patient care — the most important thing. Sarah tried her hand at hitching a ride down to the hospital via our rig. I politely told her no and prompted Jeff to get us out of there.

This book of the law shall not depart out of thy mouth; but thou shalt meditate therein day and night, that thou mayest observe to do according to all that is written therein: for then thou shalt make thy way prosperous: and then thou shalt have good success.
Joshua 1:8

#64

In-depth Incest

Paramedic Pointer» *IVs give paramedics direct access to the bloodstream via veins. The time it takes for the drugs administered to take effect is only 30-60 seconds.*

This is one of those calls that really creeped me the heck out — and it would have creeped you out too had you been there that night at 3:30 AM. I awoke from a comfortable sleep by the lovely tones in the station that invaded my inner ear — tones that would have forced even a mummy to awake from its tomb. When you're down (asleep) for a few hours during the nighttime and receive a call, a five-minute wake up period is usually appreciated. For this reason, I was happy the call location was a decent distance away from our station.

This type of family was the last thing on earth I expected to run into while my mind was still recalibrating from being in sleep mode. The emergency was for chest pain. The house we responded to was positioned on a busy street — not one of those inner neighborhood streets where one car passes per hour. The street this particular house rested on was an extremely common road for travel. Of course, the street wasn't busy on this night, seeing as though it was in the wee hours of the morning. The front porch light was on, which served as extra confirmation that Jeff and I were in the right spot. "Are you good to go?" I asked my partner Jeff as I handed him his medium-sized, purple gloves. "Yeah, I'm going to have to be," he replied with crust in the corners of his eyes. We then exited the ambulance cab and pulled our stretcher out of the back, which had each of our medical bags on it.

A black gentleman, about 40 years old, opened the door. "Can you point us to our patient?" I asked the man. I already knew, for the most part, that our patient was not him because our notes stated that the patient was both a female and 72 years old. He made no facial expression, which I thought was peculiar compared to every last one of the calls I've been on eliciting some sort of emotional response from family members. Little did I know what I'd be walking into once the eccentric black gentleman allowed us to enter. He stepped to the side and pushed the door gently to a fully open position and simply stood there looking at us. He gave a look that said, "Are you two idiots or what? Come inside before I get angry."

Right then and there I was on guard because his energy was off.

Directly into view came the 72-year-old grandma sitting on the couch. She looked pale — though she was black, her color was wan. Things appeared to be typical, as we were still surveying the scene from outside the front door. Grabbing each end of our stretcher firmly, Jeff and I advanced into our patient's living quarters. What I saw next reminded me of an episode from the X-Files — a show I watched from time to time as a child. There was an episode where murders kept occurring in a small town and the private investigators received a tip on an old abandoned house having suspicious activity. When the private investigators went to that house, they almost lost their lives because there was a serial killing, incest family who ate their victims and put them in the refrigerator to preserve uneaten portions of the bodies they killed.

Mind you, the grandma and the fellow who answered the door looked completely normal. But in that front room sat the rest of the family — adolescent children who all looked grossly deformed. Facial features seemed to be mixed and matched and out of place. Four adolescent children sat on the couch licking their lips, tapping their feet anxiously and salivating from their mouths. With all due respect to that family, I almost had to pinch myself because I thought I might have still been asleep. If only that were true I would have woke up and been so grateful because the chills running through my body gave me goose bumps along my skin.

It felt as though Jeff and I were going to be mauled to death just for being there, let alone if any of them got the false notion that we were hurting their precious grandmother. Taking a deep breath, I cleared my mind so that I could focus properly. "Hello, I'm Lorenzo and this is my partner Jeff... is it chest pain that's bothering you tonight?" I asked. "Yes darling, my chest has been aching for about 30 minutes now... it woke me up outta my sleep," grandma replied as she held the center of her chest with a bawled fist pressed against it. "I'm going to do a few things to you before we get you down to the hospital, okay?" I advised her. "Okay baby, do what you've got to do," she replied.

My partner Jeff and I began to unravel our cardiac wires and electrodes (stickers) to place on her body — we needed to get an accurate waveform, or picture of the woman's heart, to see if she was having real issues such as a heart attack or electrolyte imbalances.

Next, the strangest thing occurred — which by the way, scared the crap out of me. As I hooked grandma up to my monitor, an animal-like growl came from a back room. I could tell that it was a human, however, due to barely audible gibberish between growls. Whoever it was also sneezed. What made the unsettling growling noises worse is that the door the noises were coming from was being slammed shut. But it didn't sound as if the door was being opened wide and slammed shut; more like cracked open about an inch or two and then slammed shut. Whoever it was cracked the door open enough so that their intimidating snarls were heard, followed by a violent closing of the bedroom door. At any moment I felt as if someone was going to tackle me and start gnawing on my neck until they ate through the flesh successfully. During the process of obtaining my baseline set of vital signs and acquiring a picture of grandma's heart, my nerves bothered me more and more.

The last thing I needed to accomplish was an IV. Jeff had positioned himself behind me at this point, as if to guard the direction those horrific growls were coming from. "Thank God," I thought. "Now I can relax since he's got my back covered." I happened to glance up at the son — the initial man who opened the front door — once I finished gaining IV access on my knees. He was sitting in the corner of the room in a red suede chair, staring at me with a gaze of a psychopath who's conscience is *absent*. His legs were crossed and his general pose conveyed a psychopathic arrogance about him.

My first impression of him had been confirmed.

Something was wrong with this whole picture — I'm not sure exactly what — but something was seriously wrong. His energy was off from the start and now it felt as though that negative energy had been elevated. My gut feeling told me to get out of there — and fast! Those piercing eyes from the 40-year-old son stared me down like a lion preying on a mouse. Something told me that the only reason he didn't make a violent move was because that would jeopardize the health of his mother. He knew that I knew something wasn't right with his household and that pissed him off. The 10 minutes or so Jeff and I spent in that house felt more like an hour— uncomfortable scenarios tend to have that effect on you.

Pleased to finally be done with our diagnostics, I motioned Jeff to help me get grandma onto our gurney to get the heck out of there. A sudden rush of relief came over me in passing back through the front door on the way out to the Ambo. Grandma turned out to be having a heart attack. We ran lights and sirens to the hospital due to the severity of her biological state.

And we know that all things work together for good to them that love God, to them who are called according to his purpose.
Romans 8:28

#65

Backhoe Brainbleed

Paramedic Pointer» *When administering medication, paramedics ensure they are following the "6 rights". They are: Right patient, Right medication, Right Route (Ex. IV, oral, nasal, etc.), Right dose, Right time (expiration date) and Right documentation. These 6 rights help us practice safe treatment when giving drugs.*

I t's 9 AM in the morning on a sunny Saturday. A station in our district got selected to be leveled, station number eight, to be exact. My partner Jeff and I found it a bit strange to be responding to this location. The reason for our response was merely for a "man down" on the property, according to our computer notes. Everything was leveled at station eight when we arrived all right, including our patient. "Medic 16 on scene," Jeff keyed up the mic to tell the EMS dispatchers. All there was in the empty lot was piles of cement, a gigantic backhoe machine, and a team of construction workers gathered around a young Hispanic male lying supine on the pavement.

All of the construction workers had their hardhats on, but the young Hispanic male did not. We were literally at a demolition site. Everything from the heap of construction rubble mixed with the morning fog, making it a bit difficult to see more than my own footsteps in front of me. "We've got a

C-collar under the head of the stretcher, right?" I double checked with Jeff. A C-color is a neck brace used to keep one's head immobilized. "We sure do!" Jeff confirmed.

"Hello, what's going on this morning?" I asked the squad of construction workers as soon as we got close enough for them to hear me. The bunch of construction workers separated into two, clearing an open path to the patient. Surprisingly, the young man looked to be in pretty decent shape. "He got knocked out by that backhoe over there," someone stepped forward and exclaimed. "Knocked out? So he definitely lost consciousness?" I asked. "Yes, definitely… he was out for a good 45 seconds for sure," a man stated.

"I was?!" The Hispanic patient asked in amazement. He began to chuckle a little bit. It was a small relief to see that our patient, who had literally been knocked out, was in good spirits. "OWWW!" the patient said as he grabbed his neck. Maybe I did get knocked out…this pain is killing me!" he exclaimed. "Let's go ahead and sit you up straight if you can… do you think you can do that?" "Yes sir," the patient said. Before we sat him up right, we applied a C-collar for the protection of his neck. "This may be uncomfortable but it's for your best interest, trust me," I advised. "Yeah no problem man, I don't mind… my neck and head are killing me though!" he complained.

"Once my partner Jeff and I get you into our truck, we'll see about giving you some pain medication," I assured him. "Thanks brother… man… this pain is ridiculous, and I'm a tough guy. I used to get into fights all the time… that's what I was known for!" he boasted. In checking the back of his head, there were no gashes or any sign of head trauma. But there was a drainage coming from his right ear — it was blood. There isn't much in the prehospital setting that we do for drainage (blood or cerebral spinal fluid) from the ear other than catching it with cotton gauze pads. Jeff obtained a base set of vitals as I drew up a dosage of dilaudid for our patient's excruciating pain. "Can you tell me what city we're in, what the date is, who the president is, etc.?" I asked the patient. The whole purpose of these questions was to measure his level of orientation. He answered each of the orientation questions accurately, letting Jeff and I know that he wasn't confused. "How old are you?" Jeff asked the Hispanic male. "I'm 35 years old," he said, reaching to hold his neck. The patient's eyes became a bit heavy once I delivered the dose of dilaudid through his pipe of a vein; pain medication has a tendency to get a person feeling euphoric, which no one ever seems to complain about.

Some people reject pain medication from horror stories they hear about a family member who accepted narcotics for medical treatment. Though to my knowledge there are certainly allergic and adverse reactions that may occur (as with any drug), narcotic analgesics don't *kill* people — a common attachment to those horror stories involving pain meds. And then there are those on the opposite side of the spectrum who want everything to do with receiving pain medication because they have become addicted! They'll even go as far as to fake an injury or illness.

Our ride down to the ER was nice and smooth. No hiccups (negative surprises) arose en route to the local hospital. The ambulance roundabout at the ER — a curved hill with an awning above it specifically for emergency vehicles dropping off patients — was packed with EMS units. However, due to the severity of our patient (it being a head injury and all), Jeff and I got bumped to the front of the line once we entered the ER. Our patient's mechanism of injury (hit with a backhoe) coupled with the outcome (being knocked out) warranted a head scan on the patient.

As always, our dispatchers were hailing us to become available as soon as we made patient transfer. I gave the receiving nurse the patient's medical history, meds and allergies after disclosing what had just happened to him. My nurse's name was Talia, a real sweetheart every time I delivered patients to her — no matter how backed up she was with patients. See, similar to waitressing nurses have multiple beds to tend to all at once just as a waiter or waitress serves many tables all at the same time. Nurses do a great job of doing this, so much kudos to them for being so efficient!

Jeff and I were resetting our truck inventory and remaking our stretcher bed for the next caller as soon as I was done giving report to Talia. Later that day, when we returned, we spoke with Talia about the young Hispanic man who had been knocked out. "He ended up having a very small bleed in his brain, but he's going to be okay," Talia advised. "Is he going to have surgery then, I assume?" I replied. "No, actually, the bleed is so tiny that it is expected to heal on its own. 'The blood vessel in his brain will clot by itself,' is what the trauma surgeon told us. He will be under close monitoring, however, that's for certain," she explained.

"Wow, I never would have thought that he'd be *bypassing* surgery — but good for him! Hey, thanks again Talia, you're the best," I said with a smile as I backed away.

For whom the Lord loveth He chasteneth, and scourgeth every son whom He receiveth. If ye endure chastening, God dealeth with you as with sons; for what son is he whom the father chasteneth not? **Hebrews 12:6 – 7**

#66

The Wall That Caused It All

Paramedic Pointer» *Triage is a term used to define the prioritizing, or "sorting" of patients, based on the severity of their injuries.*

Manatee High ran an ROTC training and development course for said members from the school on this fair weathered afternoon. It was unfortunate that our instructional notes advised us of the wrong corner to enter through to get to the football field in the back of the school. We were advised to enter through the northeast gate of the high school and quickly found out that there was no gate at the northeast corner of the school. I guess what dispatch meant to put was the *southeast* corner, because that is where we found an open gateway. That minor mistake ate up an extra two minutes of response time, but mistakes happen in life.

We were told that our patient was located at the bottom of the ROTC wall — *this* information turned out to be completely accurate. I was able to snake through the open gate, just barely, with the huge ambulance. Alongside of the driver-side window was a young boy dressed in army fatigue, sprinting next to us. He took it upon himself to lead us to his downed ROTC companion. He was sweating profusely, the beady droplets glistening on his copper skin. "He's running his butt off isn't he?" I facetiously asked Jeff. There was no question about it — this young fella was running as if *his* life depended on it.

The near side of the football field had a multitude of people scattered along the straightaway on the track like salt and pepper. For this reason, Jeff and I took the long way around the track, driving around to the far side. When we came around the second curve of the 400m track, that ROTC wall was dead center in front of us. A small group of people were knelt down at the foot of the ROTC wall, tending to a small female, who looked to be mulatto. Army recruiters and other dressed out military persons were looking for ways to chip in on the general care of the young girl as we dismounted the ambulance cab. "My ankle! My ankle!" I suddenly heard the wails of the young girl. She cried and cried, leading me to believe that she fractured it — sprained it at a minimum.

A rope hung from the ROTC wall, the wall was set up such that you were to grab a hold of the rope and make contact with the wall with your feet, walking down the wall in this manner. That is the theory portion of this particular example. But as we all know, theory and application are two completely different animals. Immediately upon getting a close-up on our patient, who was sprawled out on a blue cushioned mat, I recognized that one ankle was extremely more swollen than the other. "Can you grab a pillow out of the truck please?" I asked my partner Jeff. There was a gentleman holding our patient's injured ankle up off the ground and I wanted to replace *him* with a pillow. "Oh my gosh! Oh my gosh! Where is Haley? Has anyone seen my best friend Haley?! Oh my gosh, where's my phone?!" the mulatto high school student panicked. It never ceases to amaze me how certain people are worried about everything they shouldn't be. She was so frantic and jittery about contacting her best friend that I'm not sure if her tears were for her actual injury. People are something. I've even had certain patients ask if they could take a few more puffs on their cigarette before we transported them to the ER.

"Oh my gosh, Haley!" she cried out in distress. "Can Haley come with me to the hospital?! Where's my phone?! I need to call my uncle and let him know what's going on!" This girl was a real train wreck. I'll give it to her, she was only a 15-year-old high schooler but good grief, the fact that she had 1 million concerns outside of her ankle fracture earned her the label: drama queen. "What's your name sweetheart?" I abruptly asked her name. "Cassandra," she responded through short sniffles. "Hey Cassandra, me and my partner are here to help you, but we need you to do your best to calm down… you're worried about everything under the sun right now; it's only making things worse. We're gonna bandage your fractured ankle and give you a shot of morphine okay?" I calmly explained. I tried to relay my message to her with as calm of a demeanor as possible so that she would calm down — it didn't work.

"Oh my gosh! A shot! I hate needles! You don't really have to give me a shot do you?!" she cried in a fit of acute fear. "Cassandra… listen to me, the IV I start on you won't hurt nearly as much as your broken ankle… it's going to be a pinch. And you'll thank me for it later when the morphine kicks in," I stated. "Awww okay… fine," she reluctantly accepted. "Hold still and whatever you do, don't flinch when I poke you," I cautioned Cassandra. "I won't," she said through a couple of involuntary sniffles. Jeff placed her injured ankle softly on the pillow he grabbed from the truck and began wrapping a Sam Splint (immobilization board for extremities) around her ankle to keep it stable. "Here we go… big poke… ready?" I tricked her into thinking I cared whether or not she was actually ready because by the time she actually opened her mouth to reply, the IV was already done.

"All done!" I uttered quickly. "All we have to do is get you lifted onto our stretcher and then you can just sit back and relax — no more moving for you until we get to the ER. "… okay" Cassandra reluctantly whined. I lifted Cassandra's upper body by placing my arms under her armpits. Jeff lifted her legs while we designated a military recruiter to specifically maintain manual stabilization of her fractured ankle. The rest of the ROTC students clapped as we placed Cassandra on our cot and began to buckle her in. "How long do you think they'll keep me there?" Cassandra asked once we loaded her into the truck. "It's a good chance that they'll release you once you receive a cast and crutches for that ankle," I replied. "Okay, great because I hate hospitals…

they're so boring." Arriving at the ER marked the cessation of our time spent with Cassandra. The receiving nurse took report from me and signed my transfer of care documentation. Cassandra never did figure out where her best friend Haley was, but Cassandra, herself, found herself to be right where she needed to be.

For the Lord loveth judgment, and forsaketh not His saints; they are preserved forever: but the seed of the wicked shall be cut off.
Psalm 37:28

#67

Mental Group Home

Paramedic Pointer» *Happiness is defined by the one in pursuit of it. The nature of your mentality sets the stage for your own success. Like the bible says, "For as he thinketh in his heart, so is he (or she)."*

This job introduces the cold hard truth to not only paramedics, but nearly anyone working in the medical field. From the rich neighborhoods to the dingy ghettos, we see all walks of life. There is no age limit to injury and illness. Nor is there a prejudice misfortune has against anyone. *No one* is immune to sickness and/or injuries.

I'd like to take the time out to tell of a group home that housed nothing but special needs individuals — specifically the mentally challenged. As a Christian, it was always a struggle to grasp the fact that God allows certain humans to be born with a handicap or decreased sense of mentation. I often think to myself, "Why was I born normal while another person has some birth defect he or she could not control?" And further, "Whatever happened to free will? If God gives us free will, why don't we have the decision to be born perfectly healthy or choose how we will look?" There are two things I have concluded in that line of questioning: God is in control of what he creates and secondly, things aren't always as bad as they may seem. I'll explain to you exactly what I mean.

When you merely glance at a mentally disabled person, one of the first thoughts that may cross your mind is, "What a difficult life to live… filled with struggle and limitations." But my experience at a response to a mental group home showed me another side to the coin.

"These people are going to love you Lorenzo… one of the women are always hitting on me when I come here," Jeff exclaimed with a laugh. An employee opened the entrance door to let us through. Just inside, in the front dining room sat a number of residents eating their supper. It was about 6:45 PM and they were having a ball! There was so much laughter in the air as the residents mumbled about Lord knows what, amongst themselves.

One of the mentally challenged residents had a slew of drool dribbling down the corner of her mouth. Her friend, seated directly next to her, uttered, "You are so silly… you're such a silly girl!" As she took a napkin and dabbed the saliva from the woman's mouth. There was a keen sense of family they exemplified in being sure to let us know that Eleanor (our patient) needed our help. They were also eager to help Jeff and I get going in the right direction and also help one another. I could see and feel the honest love they had for one another as friends. And it got me thinking, "These people are not sitting around wondering why they aren't like everyone else. Heck, they may not even be aware that they aren't exactly like everyone else in terms of their mental capabilities." Seeing this showed me that everything isn't what it seems. These people were having a great time! In fact, I hadn't seen this much honest laughter since my childhood at the school playground!

Eleanor, our patient, was waiting for us in her room—she was as relaxed as she could be. "What's wrong with Ms. Eleanor today?" I asked her nurse. —"NOTHING!" Eleanor butted in to the conversation. I began to crack a smile, but kept my composure in waiting for the nurse's response. "She hasn't been breathing normal today. Her oxygen saturation reading was low when I checked it earlier," the Caucasian nurse explained. Eleanor seemed to be doing just fine, no apparent difficulty breathing just by looking at her. I unwrapped my stethoscope from around my neck and pressed it against Eleanor's chest to listen for lung sounds. No abnormal breath sounds were heard. No wheezes. No rhonchi. No Stridor (All abnormal lung sounds). And certainly, no fluid bubbling about in her lungs. "How do you feel Ms. Eleanor?" I asked in a loud tone accompanied by a smile. "I don't want to go to the hospital!" Eleanor announced with no further delay of her desired outcome.

Eleanor was a 78-year-old Caucasian female. She was as cute as a button — one could mistake her for a child from her playful demeanor and flamboyant personality. "She seems to be breathing just fine to me," I stated respectfully. "Her doctor wants her to be transported, we just spoke on the phone," Eleanor's nurse told me. "Aha", I thought. "The old over-the-phone diagnosis." "Okay no problem... we'll take her on down to be evaluated." Jeff had just finished up acquiring a baseline set of vitals when I said to Eleanor, "Hey dear... I know you want to stay home, but we're gonna have to take you anyway, hun, okaaay?" "AWWWW!" Eleanor moaned. Even though she didn't want to go, she maintained a jolly old grin on her face. "AWWWW... okkaaayy..." Eleanor continued. There wasn't much at all to be done to Eleanor outside of general monitoring on the way to the ER. Her transport was completely precautionary.

Nonetheless, it allowed me to broaden my perspective on the disabled. Just because a person faces challenges in life doesn't mean they aren't happy. If you ever find yourself pondering the intentions of what God allows to happen just remember: God is the potter and we are the clay — he is in control. And I'm not just telling you these things to sound positive — he really *is* in control. He took me from situations that were indeed hell in a hand basket and placed me in much better positions. You can learn about many accounts of how God worked in my life from my debut book, *The Corridor That Lies Between Greatness and Insanity*. But in short, I will tell you I've gone from workplace hell to workplace heaven. I've been given tangible, visible signs, that God is real. I've experienced great healing from heartbreak. Whatever your dilemmas are, God can heal. Whenever you're forced to bend, remember that God can *mend*. Take care of yourself. I'll meet you at the next tale.

For if a man think himself to be something, when he is nothing, he deceiveth himself. **Galatians 6:3**

#68

The Same Old Drunk

Paramedic Pointer» *Alcohol is the most widely abused drug in the United States. More than 100 million Americans regularly consume alcohol. Alcoholism remains one of the top five causes of death in the United States.*

"What are you doing out here, Steve?" I yelled. The homeless man wearing a faded green ball cap, carrying bags, took one look at me and brushed me off. I was hanging just outside the sliding side door of the ambulance, hoping Steve had a legit reason for dialing 911. See, me and Steve are well acquainted. Every third day (on my day of duty), Steve got someone to let him use the telephone at the local CVS store. The funny thing about it was that Steve was so punctual with his call from CVS. Every single time he called it was at 9:00 PM, likely the time he needed a comfy place to sleep and a meal—a place like the hospital. Which is as good as a five-star hotel when you're homeless.

"I see Steve more than I see my own darn family!" snarled Jeff. I had grown tired of transporting the same guy, but Jeff was on another level with his weariness. He was completely fed up. Just like any other service, EMS is not perfect. Like many other systems, there are loopholes— loopholes where people can misuse the system. In this particular line of work, we refer to it as 911 *abuse*. Poor Jeff let Steve get under his skin so bad one time that he nearly lost control, grabbing Steve by the collar and saying, "Look... I'm tired of dealing with your crap... don't call us unless you need us! There are people out here that genuinely need our help... unlike you!"

Of course I had a chat with Jeff about it and he agreed that it was a bit unprofessional. He had a point though. There have been instances where homeless people have been far away from their fort and decided to call an ambulance when it was going to rain. It's a real shame but it happens. And in our system, we can't refuse anyone who expresses a need to go to the hospital — even if they have no means to pay the bill. But homeless people don't care about a bill anyhow — there's no address or real account anywhere to tax!

Speaking of ambulance bills, they are absolutely horrendous. I'll even go as far as to say that they are unscrupulous. Try $500 – $600 for a transport to the ER. A word to the wise: EMS is a wonderful service to have when you absolutely need it — did I mention *only* when you absolutely need it? Be sure that you are using good judgment when utilizing an ambulance ride, because you will be charged handsomely — unless of course you're someone like Steve. The reason why Steve tried to shrug me off when he saw me was because this was likely the fifth time now that we'd be transporting him — he knew Jeff and I were on to his scheme. So the look he gave me said, "Oh no... not this guy again... he knows my agenda." Steve began walking away with his gimpy leg. Steve did have a chronic swelling in his left foot that he wore a compression cast on. On his left foot was his compression boot and on his right was an old brown colored flip-flop that must have been found in a filthy dumpster.

Though Steve's swollen foot was authentic, it was old news. And not to mention, the bigger issue here was Steve's chronic alcohol abuse/addiction. Alcohol was where Steve's true problem lied. The poor guy couldn't sober up long enough to do something that actually made sense — like be productive. "Come on over here Steve," I called to him. He slowed down to a standstill and began to briefly plan his next move. "Heyyy..." he squinted his eyes at me. "Do I know you?" he continued. Steve decided to play dumb, as if him acting like he didn't know me would somehow make me forget that I knew *him*. "Yes I know you, don't play games with me tonight," I warned him. Shamelessly continuing on with his plan, he said, "Really...? Well then where do I know you from?" he tried to be witty. "Your name is Steve, you love the *Redskins*, you drink nothing but vodka — no beer — and you like to go to the hospital for your chronic swollen foot," I fired off.

Steve shot me a mile-wide grin as if to say, "You got me." "Well hot dog you son of a gun, you do know me!" he began to laugh. "Anyone who knows me knows I stay away from beer! I'm a vodka man, ha!" "Do you need to go to the hospital tonight?" I asked. "Yeah man, my foot is killing me, but they always just send me home," he complained. "Yes I know; that's because there's nothing they can do for that swollen foot at this point. And they're going to do the same thing tonight — send you right to the fast track department and out the door! But I can't deny you a transport if you want to go so what's it going to be?"

He thought about it for a few seconds and said, "My foot really is killing me man… there's gotta be something they can do." "Get inside the rig, Steve," I told him. These calls are certainly not the ones paramedics live for. Individuals like Steve should be tagged by society as *time wasters*. One local hospital did so by banning Steve from their facility, marking him as a trespasser. Now all Jeff and I needed was for the other hospitals to do the same.

But He was wounded for our transgressions, He was bruised for our iniquities: the chastisement of our peace was upon Him; and with His stripes we are healed. **Isaiah 53:5**

#69

The Last Ditch Effort

Paramedic Pointer» The CNS (Central Nervous System) is made up of the brain and the spinal cord. The brain is the main data center of the body, consisting of the cerebrum (regulates higher-level functioning such as thought) and the cerebellum (which maintains coordination).

Have you ever been between a rock and a hard place, so to speak? And all you were given was one last battle cry, before all the walls caved in on you? This is what they refer to as a *last ditch effort* — but you knew that already. Let's talk about that saying's origins. Maybe that's something you don't happen to know. Allegedly the old phrase comes from historic military terminology from William III when he told his soldiers to "Fight until the bitter end in the last ditch." In other words, "Give it all you've got because it may be your last chance to do so."

In the broad world of EMS responses, the last ditch effort we paramedics come across ironically have nothing to do with medical or traumatic emergencies — not authentically anyway. People will do some petty things when their back is against the wall — like lie. There have been teenage girls arrested for shoplifting and just before getting hauled off to jail suddenly have this mysterious chest pain or shortness of breath. Other times people call to get trivial abrasions (scrapes) assessed to stall for time — quite possibly to plan an escape. I've actually responded to the police station where they had the criminals in a line, being checked in at registration. One of them got us to evaluate him and demanded to be seen at an ER, knowing that we legally couldn't reject his request. On his way out the jail's front doors, he looked over at one of his criminal homeboys and winked at him. His buddy winked back and began to give a supportive laugh as if to say, "You go boy."

A scrawny woman named Teresa stands out in my mental archive when I think of one of those last ditch efforts. Teresa was stopped by the police at approximately 2:15 AM. It turns out that she was driving without a license. In fact, her license had been revoked, so it made no difference whether she had it or not. One thing I have to give a person like Teresa credit for is the fact that she had an entertaining excuse for as to why she was out and about without legal permission to be behind the wheel.

"I was on the way to the ER to get my forearm checked out... it's been swelling up bigger and bigger the past few days." The only problem with this tall tale from Teresa was that it was more than evident that she was a drug addict. Her speech and mannerisms betrayed her. And the multiple holes in her arms from "shooting up" explained the swelling that was almost the size of a standard light bulb in her forearm. What really caused her forearm swelling was the fact that she missed the vein when she tried to start her own IV line. Jeff and I always chuckle when a patient treats us as if it's our first day. Give me a break. The wise guys and wise gals are forever thinking that *they* are the exception. As if they are the one and only unseen glitch in the system that will go unnoticed.

We escorted Teresa to the side of the ambulance — this was the easier means of getting inside the truck due to an extra step that electronically deployed just above the ground when you opened the ambulance sliding door. Teresa sat down and vanished deeper into what she thought was incognito; her acting skills of playing the injured damsel in distress were riveting — until of course she came upon the startling realization that her award-winning acting didn't *undo* her crime. After we turned the second corner, or so, from leaving the scene, Teresa squinted her eyes, peering out the back windows of the ambulance.

"Heyyyy… Why are the police behind us? Are they following us?!" she shrugged in grave disappointment. "Yes, they're going to link up with you again at the hospital," I replied. "Ugh…what for? I just got done talking to them!" "According to what one of the cops told me, you were out driving when you weren't supposed to be and you have a warrant out for your arrest." Teresa simply sat quietly in her blue jeans and torn brown T-shirt. She already knew everything that I had just told her. But she thought she had successfully flown under the radar somehow. Teresa was monitored until transfer of care was made at the ER. Following her medical evaluation to ensure her medical clearance, she would be taken to jail— as originally planned— when she was pulled over.

To Him give all the prophets witness, that through His name whosoever believeth in him shall receive remission of sins. **Acts 10:43**

#70

Attack The Asthma

Paramedic Pointer» *3 things occur with the presentation of asthma, they are referred to as the "Asthma Triad": 1) Airway Edema (swelling) 2) Bronchospasm (airway gets smaller) and 3) Increased mucus production*

Suffocation isn't a pleasant experience; not being able to breathe causes panic, confusion, damage to the heart and brain — and ultimately death. Some of us have experienced being drowned almost, by that childhood playmate that couldn't swim and decided to use us as a buoy — shoving you down to stay afloat or strangling you while trying to avoid sinking. Now, I mentioned that example to mention this: that kind of occurrence is likely a one or two-time happening, only to be lost in our minds as trivial encounters over time. But imagine if they weren't a fluke experience you had once or twice. Let's say you experienced that kind of devastating lack of oxygen on a frequent basis, so much that you were required to carry around a device to save you when those times come around. Let's take it one step further: so you had that life saving device on you at all times, but ran out of the medication the device is filled with by mistake. What I'm describing to you is the life of a person diagnosed with asthma. One lady, who had lived with asthma for years, had a bout with it that could have taken her life.

She was an old woman, located in the heart of a mobile home community just outside of zone 16; Jeff and I ended up having to cover for another unit that was bogged down with calls. Not nearly as familiar with this zone as our own beloved zone 16 (I say beloved sarcastically), Jeff and I took the time to thoroughly study our map on the way to the call. In doing so, we still managed to pass our patient's house by a few feet. Coming to a screeching halt once we realized we had gone one house too far, Jeff kicked it in reverse and backed up a few feet. "Here you go," I said to Jeff, handing him a pair of medium, purple gloves to save some time. We knew that our patient was experiencing difficulty breathing, we just didn't know to what extent. But our female's appearance and posture said it all once we got a good look at her. She was as pale as a ghost with a hint of cyanosis (blue-tinted skin), sitting in the tripod position.

The tripod position is an attempt to align one's airway axis, done by sitting down with both hands on one's knees while leaning forward. She was at a loss for words — literally; to our fortune, her husband was home to aid us with some useful information. "Maggie is my wife... she's got asthma... she ran out of her medication for her metered-dose inhaler," he exclaimed. "Please get her back to normal guys... I don't want to lose her!" he elevated his voice with worry.

"I CAN'T BREATHE! I CAN'T BREATHE!" cried Maggie, who looked to be about 80 years old. "Don't worry Miss Maggie, you're in good hands," I assured her as Jeff and I began to intervene. Maggie was wearing an ivory, satin nightgown. She was barefoot and her hair was drenched in the sweat she had worked up from fighting to breathe. She must have owned about five cats, or so, because they were everywhere; I kept having to watch my step to avoid tripping down. I cringed every time one of the cats grazed across my pant leg because I'm ridiculously allergic to cats — Jeff as well. Jeff broke out the oxygen tank and nebulizer to prepare a breathing treatment filled with the same medication Maggie was already on. *Albuterol* and *Atrovent*, probably the most common asthma drugs, dilate the airway in order for the patient to breathe. What happens in an asthma attack is the opposite of dilation — constriction — leaving one short of breath and wheezing their brains out. That same airway constriction is what causes those wheezes.

"I CAN'T BREATHE! I CAN'T BREATHE!" Maggie muttered as she grasped the arm of the sofa she was sitting on with both hands. "We've got oxygen coming right up Miss Maggie… we're getting your breathing treatment ready now," I told her with empathy. Maggie began to shake ever so slightly— her shaking resembled shivers. "Okay Miss Maggie, here's some oxygen for you," I said while pulling the oxygen mask over her pale face. "It's important that we get you on to our stretcher hun…that way we can get you on down to the hospital… can you stand and sit right back down on the stretcher?" I asked. I had positioned the cot such that all she had to do was stand and pivot onto it with ease.

Maggie attempted to stand up and it only resulted in her plopping back down in the same spot. Jeff put the nebulizer down, which was now loaded with medication, to help me lift her onto the cot. (A nebulizer is a medical device that mystifies liquid medications for breathing such as Albuterol and Atrovent). "Aanndd…up we go!" Jeff chanted in lifting her off of the sofa. —PLOP! It was a quick and dirty transfer from her couch to our stretcher. Glancing at her oxygen saturation levels on the cardiac monitor, I could gather that her reading was very low. "Let's get some medication going! Pass me the nebulizer!" I urged Jeff. He passed it to me one second later.

"Okay Miss Maggie, you know the drill… breathe in as deep as you can and hold it in! Repeat this over and over until the medication has all disappeared!" I coached her. Maggie now held the nebulizer in her mouth on her own; Jeff and I packed up our medical bags and expedited exiting the residence. Maggie sucked down the misty medication like she had never breathed before. "Very good Miss Maggie! You'll be back to normal in no time! Keep up the great work, you're doing awesome," I encouraged her. In little time, Maggie's color had already started returning. Her violent, labored breathing throttled back considerably as well. Things were looking up! "I think we're good back here Lorenzo," Jeff said as I finished her IV and blood pressure in the rear of the ambulance.

Jeff and I alternate driving to the hospital. It was my turn to be the driver. "Sounds good to me, I'll see you at the hospital Miss Maggie!" I said before closing the back doors. She shook her head up and down, trying earnestly to still retain as much of the nebulized medication as possible. This particular mobile home community was a gigantic maze. If you don't pay close attention to the computer map in places like these, one wrong turn can leave you lost or going in circles. There was an important turn to make in order to get back to the community's exit gates — I made sure I didn't miss it. On the way out I saw multiple elderly folks wearing those huge black sunglasses that could block the sun even if it was only one mile away. They were just wandering around, enjoying the weather; a few of the community residents were walking their dogs or bending corners in their golf carts. But I kid you not, all of them had their handy sunglasses on — you'd think they came with x-ray vision or something due to how bulky they are!

When we arrived at the ER, I scurried around to the rear of the rig to dismount Miss Maggie from the ambulance — I was anxious to see if she'd gotten better or worse over the 10 minutes of transport time. To say the least, I was greatly pleased to find that Miss Maggie looked like a million bucks! "Hey! You're looking brand-new now aren't you?" I said excitedly. "Yes… I feel much better now… I thought that was the end for me." Maggie stated. "How could it be the end for you? You have such a dynamic duo helping you today!" I replied. "Because I couldn't breathe! Wow…what a scary feeling! I was sure that God was ready for me to come home!" she said. "Not today Miss Maggie, today is not your day for that…hope you're not disappointed," I joked.

She gave me a big smile and proceeded to puff on the nebulizer a few short puffs at a time. "Once we get you inside, a doctor will come check you out; they'll draw some blood from you and check out your overall status." "Okay" she responded. The nurse was happy to see Miss Maggie doing so well when placing her in the ER bed — since we fixed the problem, all the receiving nurse had to do was monitor for the most part. Nurses enjoy that luxury when they can get it. Asthma comes around every so often looking for a victim to attack. My partner and I show up to deal with these conflicts with the intent to defuse the issue. Today we showed up to attack asthma — and we won.

Therefore if any man be in Christ, he is a new creature: old things are passed away; behold, all things are become new. **2 Corinthians 5:17**

71

A Pleasant Awakening

Paramedic Pointer» *There is two types of Diabetics, they are referred to as "Type 1" or "Type 2". In type 1, most patients do not produce insulin and it typically develops in childhood. In type 2, the person becomes dependent on insulin. Diabetes is the #1 cause for blindness.*

Two of my favorite kinds of calls are diabetic patients and overdose patients. Being a results-driven individual, these two particular calls excite me the most because there is typically a lightning-fast turnaround time from being unconscious to being alert. Diabetic patients can become severely *hypoglycemic* (low blood sugar) and in turn, become unresponsive. Since the blood sugar is so low, their mentation drops too because the brain needs sugar to function properly. As for overdose patients, dangerous drugs like heroin decrease breathing rates and mentation as well — leaving the user comatose. But what I love so much is that their return (both diabetics and overdosers) to consciousness is so speedy— almost instant— with the help of our amazing drugs. A lot of overdose patients wake up highly pissed off and ready to fight. But why, if their lives have just been saved?

It's because they *aren't* worried about their life being preserved — otherwise they wouldn't be doing the heroin in the first place. No, they're worried about achieving their high, and it pisses them off when they realize the money they blew on achieving that high has been blown in an instant by a caring EMS worker. Diabetics respond much differently when they are revived, so to speak. In fact, a gentleman had such an epiphany when he realized that we had saved him that he couldn't contain himself!

Around 1:15 AM, Jeff and I received notification from our station intercom. First the ear stabbing emergency tones sounded off, followed by the electronic woman's voice, "Medic 16…respond on TAC 4 for diabetic complications." My bladder was full of, well, you know what it was full of, but there was no time to use the restroom because we had to get going. Zipping up my jumpsuit, I rushed out to the truck and hopped in. It was quiet darkness tonight — Jeff and I cruised down the freeway rather peacefully. The nice thing about no one being on the road is that you can bypass using the sirens, which is nice to do without for a change. Hearing the sirens every single call can get old!

The neighborhood we responded to was impressive. Nothing but nice, well-kept homes lined the streets of this classy subdivision. A Chinese woman waved us down, she was wearing a black satin robe. "Good evening Miss, what's going on tonight?" "Ehh…" she began. She then shook her head in frustration and pointed at her house, making out that someone was sleeping inside by putting her hands together and pressing them against her cheek while closing her eyes. She then frantically turned and ran inside. Jeff and I speedily grabbed our gear and resumed advancing up the driveway. "We can fit the stretcher all the way inside, I'm sure. I can tell by looking at the layout," I explained to Jeff after poking my head inside the front door for a brief moment.

Making our way through the living room, we noticed highly decorated walls with that of their culture — namely samurai swords. They were mounted on all of the walls, the family was clearly collectors. Entering the back bedroom brought into focus a Chinese man sprawled out on a king-sized bed. Like his wife, he was wearing a black satin robe. Three firemen were already on the scene and they gave us a brief, but useful report on the patient. "We just checked his blood sugar and its 19." To give the reader an idea of how low that actually is, note that normal ranges are from around 70 to 120. Our patient had no choice but to be comatose with a reading that low! "We're not sure how long he's been unconscious, but we do know that he has a history of diabetes and high blood pressure." I was already hooking him up to our cardiac monitor and wrapping the blood pressure cuff around his upper arm as the fireman spoke. "Hand me a tourniquet and a 20-gauge IV, Jeff," I requested. It was show time — my favorite part about being a paramedic — the part where I inject someone with a life-saving vial and see them return spontaneously.

The Chinese man had decent veins to work with but they were a little flat, which meant I would have to be cautious when threading the needle because there wasn't that much spare room inside the blood vessel to work with. "Here goes," I thought to myself before penetrating his skin. —STICK! In went the 20-gauge needle. A second or two after penetration with the needle, I saw a small amount of venous blood return into the chamber of my IV catheter — this meant that the IV was good. "Quick, hand me the ampule of *Dextrose*!" I requested of Jeff. He quickly pushed some of the medication out of the top to evacuate any residual air in the ampule. It's important to do this when administering medications because the last thing you want to do is push air into a patient's vein — that can cause serious complications and even kill someone.

I grabbed the ampule from Jeff and screwed it into the IV access point. I pushed the entire ampule into the unconscious Chinese man and hung a liter of fluids to help the syrup-like medication mix into the bloodstream easier. Also, I had to ensure that his blood pressure maintained at a normal level. Then we waited. The Chinese man's wife looked at each one of the EMS personnel in the room, including me. She wasn't quite sure what was going on because we had all stopped moving about for a moment and sort of just went silent. Her eyes quickly scanned each of our faces as we waited patiently for her husband to wake back up.

Suddenly the Chinese man's eyes opened slowly and he began blinking as if his brain was recalibrating. That drug having entered his blood stream flipped the reset switch in his body and now he was rebooting. He turned his head towards me — still laying down — and said, "Heyyy…you saved me!" letting out a long sigh, following his statement. "I know myself again! I know my wife!" he stated in his extremely pronounced Chinese accent. "Thank you-thank! Thank you so much!" he said with his mouth open and eyes wide open. He had experienced some sort of revelation; for he went on to speak of how he knew his name again and exactly where he was. We all laughed at his comical remarks — it was a laugh of *relief* that we had saved another patient.

Our patient was covered in sweat as he still lay flat on his back in that king-sized bed covered in plush black satin. Sitting him up, I took a towel and wiped him down, starting with his forehead. "Oh wow, I can't thank you guys enough!" he continued to show gratitude towards us all. His wife left and returned with a tall glass of ice water, her face overwhelmed with happiness. Nothing else needed to be done for the gentleman besides having him eat something to maintain his blood glucose with the dextrose (liquid sugar) we administered. He ate a peanut butter and jelly sandwich while we were still there and we checked his blood sugar again. Not wanting to go to the hospital, he asked to sign a refusal of transport. I allowed him to stay home since he was *back to earth* as they say. He thanked us and thanked us some more, all the way until his wife saw us out the door with a huge grin on her face.

For the Lord God is a sun and shield: the Lord will give grace and glory: no good thing will He withhold from them that walk uprightly. Oh Lord of hosts, Blessed is the man that trusteth in Thee. **Psalm 84:11 – 12**

#72

Autopulse Malfunction

Paramedic Pointer» *Becoming CPR certified is affordable and readily available. Hospitals and local schools offer classes all over. Become CPR certified to make yourself a powerful ally to those in need. It is both beneficial to yourself and others!*

EMS is an ever-changing machine. Constant updates on medical devices and innovative designs keep us paramedics having to stay continually educated via training courses. It's quite comical to hear how behind on things the general public is on EMS procedures. The question that comes up probably the most — even today — is: "Do you all still do mouth-to-mouth on your patients?" To answer that common inquiry: mouth-to-mouth has been done away with for some time now — it's just unsanitary. No paramedic, or anyone for that matter, wants to catch a disease while trying to save a life. What we use is masks that serve as a safe barrier between persons, a mask that we connect to a squeezable oxygen reservoir we refer to as a *bag valve mask.*

Now that I've cleared the air on that frequently asked question, I want to talk about an innovative device that will change the way we do CPR — in the sense that we *won't* be doing CPR. Yes, CPR will still be achieved, just not manually. The device I speak of is called the Autopulse. It's roughly

$15,000 – $18,000 currently and does automatic compressions with a nifty circumferential band that encompasses one's thoracic region (chest region). It revolutionizes cardiac arrest calls because instead of using up one pair of hands for manual compressions, that would-be compressor is now free to draw up drugs, control the patient's airway, start an IV, etc.

When the auto pulse first arrived at my department, every news station in my local area had to have a story on it. Jeff and I were the paramedics from my department to demonstrate it on television, and since there were three or four news crews, we did the same demonstration plenty of times. We became gurus on this new device in a matter of one day — if only that meant we would never experience difficulties with it. Our station was the first to receive this awesome innovation because we were the busiest truck in the whole county. Not long would we have to wait to use it in real time.

The stroke of 4:05 PM marked the latest cardiac arrest patient that day in zone 16. Everyone was hanging outside of a dirty liquor store in the ghetto, drinking their booze and telling lies to one another—you know, the typical tipsy trash talk. The hardcore drinkers decided to kick off their weekend a bit early, for it was a Thursday. Our fire crew had beaten us to the scene. Pulling up to the run down liquor joint, I saw the veiny forearms of a black fireman performing compressions on a downed black male with gray hair. This was going on in a parking lot made predominantly of dirt. "He's in cardiac arrest, don't forget the Autopulse," Jeff reminded me. The handles on the outside of the auto pulse carrying case are positioned in the middle so that you can carry it like a shield. I felt like a military soldier hauling the Autopulse over to the patient in that manner.

Throwing the Autopulse on the ground to be unzipped for use, one of the three firemen on scene said nervously, "Uhhh…I've never used that thing before." "Don't worry about it, I've got it covered," I replied quickly. Keep in mind that a man is clinically dead right now, CPR is in progress, and the entire parking lot posse had come over to enjoy the show. There was no shortage of spectators, increasing the suspense of our emergency call up another notch. "Come on back to us Freddy…come on back to us," a black man wearing a white wife beater cheered. He had a deep, soulful voice that sent vibrations through the air with his bass. A beer occupied his hand just like all the other onlookers. "We're gonna strap the Autopulse on our patient and let it do some work for us," I told the three firemen. "We just need to roll the patient on his side so I can scoot the device under him." "You got it," they all replied, beginning to roll him that instant.

The Autopulse had a circumferential band that was made of elastic material; it meshed together by way of velcro. Securing the band tightly around our patient's chest, I pressed the green button, which began automatic compressions. Excitement overwhelmed me, for I was happy to be running my first call with hands-free CPR! And then Murphy's Law happened— my jaw dropped. Everyone's jaw dropped. Remember that velcro/elastic band I mentioned a minute ago? Yeah, well that popped off! The manner in which it popped off was so dramatic too, which made it even more awkward and noticeable to everyone spectating. The velcro, as it came undone, made an extremely loud noise in the process and then all of a sudden…—POP!! "The life band came loose!" A fireman shouted.

I frantically intervened, connecting the band's two halves together again. "Whew!" I gasped. We made haste to load the patient on our stretcher — our handy Autopulse doing high-quality CPR throughout that transition from the dirt terrain to up on our gurney. Then again, just as we lifted the patient up to slide him into the rear of the truck, the velcro band popped off for a second time; everyone watching gasped. How bad of timing could it have been? Here we are in front of a large group of people, and our life-saving equipment is all over the place, making loud noises, popping off of our patient and such!

Instead of us looking like a bunch of heroes, we were looking more like a bunch of *zeros* at this point. Continuing into the back of the rig as smoothly as possible, I quickly closed the doors behind us. "Thank goodness," I thought. The atrocity that had occurred twice now was no longer in the public eye. "This Autopulse device isn't working! Back to manual CPR!!" I demanded. All of two seconds went by in removing the Autopulse from the patient. Uninterrupted CPR is paramount to positive patient outcomes; we are taught to not stop compressions for more than 10 seconds when assessing a pulse.

The black gentleman's eyes were sealed shut. I pulled both of his eyelids open gently with my thumbs to find that they were constricted — a sign of a likely overdose. Pressing the charge button, I looked at everyone and said, "Everyone clear yourselves!" Everybody threw their hands up, giving me the go ahead to send a powerful current of electricity through the patient. — ZZZZTTT! Our patient's body jolted violently. The black man's arm flew into the air, almost knocking Jeff out cold. The fireman doing CPR had 1 foot on the ambulance countertop and his 2nd foot on the ambulance floor. He was positioned such that he could deliver the most powerful compressions possible — sweat dripping from his brow all the while.

"Do we have a pulse?! Stop compressions!!" I directed. The aggressive fireman stopped abruptly, taking his foot off the ambulance countertop to stand firmly on two feet as he assessed our patient's neck with his index and middle fingers. "Yes…yes we do!" he looked up and announced as if he had won the prize money on a scratch off. "Hang a liter of fluid!" I urged. The black patient didn't regain consciousness on our watch, but he did survive. Even though our innovative Autopulse embarrassed us and inconvenienced our flow slightly, we still managed to save a man's life. Mistakes can be avoided at times, but if you keep going, sometimes fortune can still fall in your favor.

If any of you lack wisdom, let him ask of God, that giveth to all men liberally, and upbraideth not; and it shall be given him.
James 1:5

#73

Record Skip

Paramedic Pointer» *There are four types of distinguished skull fractures: 1)Linear, 2)Depressed, 3)Basilar and 4) Open. Head injuries most commonly occur from deceleration in motor vehicle collisions and falls.*

Today music is listened to by way of bluetooth or some sort of MP3 device. But back when people used to buy CDs, or even further back in time — records — a track was liable to skip if it was damaged. Late one night, a wave of nostalgia occurred that brought to mind the way this used to happen.

Saturday night was the precise night it was. Darkness fell over the city as softly as a comforter does when its handler fluffs it over the mattress. The quietness of our shift was disrupted and dismantled by the wiles of party animals and feuding families…oh the joys of the weekend. Everybody is trying to make the most of their two days off from their 9 to 5's, filling their time with music, television, alcohol and pure drama. People like to party, but I believe it's a whole new level when Mexicans are the ones doing the partying. From stop sign to stop sign on the neighborhood street our call was on, cars were lined up along the sides. It was late December; many houses on the block still had their Christmas lights still on, so the entire street was lit up.

Our call was located on the right hand side of that car-filled street, just as the straightaway turned into a curve. A sea of policemen were standing together, bunched up like a swarm of bees as they vigorously consulted with one another. It was 2:30 AM. Though I was still trying to wake up fully, it didn't take long. All of the brilliant christmas lights mixed with the police cars, firetruck and ambulance lights flickering all at once, forced my eyes open. I was wondering whether to ask if someone had disco music because it looked like we had been in some sort of disco party. Jeff and I walked up to the slew of policemen and asked if the scene was secure; before this, all we knew was that a male patient was physically assaulted. "The scene is clear, the suspect fled the scene. We were told by a family member that the patient was hit with a bat. That is what allegedly caused the trauma", he finished.

Jeff and I exchanged serious looks and hurriedly advanced towards the backyard of the home. The stretcher wheels are plenty durable; they're just not that big, so when we rolled through an area filled with dirt, we met great resistance. We had to shift our efforts into a higher gear and pull extra hard to get our cot as close as possible to our patient. He was a very short man—about 5 feet even—lying face down in the dirt. Just as a person's face would sink into a pie if they laid their face in one, this man's face was sunk down into the *earth*—it was a mud pie. The back of his head had blood running from a gaping hole that looked like a meteor crashed into it. The darkness kept me from being able to discern whether his blood was a dark red or purplish color. "Do you have a flashlight on you Jeff?" I asked. Without words, he took an LED flashlight out of his cargo pocket and handed it over to me — still looking on at the patient in awe.

—CLICK-CLICK! Suddenly the flashlight lit up almost the whole backyard and we were able to see. The back of the man's head was caved in with blood bubbling out of the crater the baseball bat created. First things first. We had to get his face out of the dirt so that his airway was clear. Jeff held his head steady and I rallied two firemen to help me roll the patient's body so that he was lying face up on his back. "Ayyye...ayyye..." the short Mexican man murmured. "What is your name sir?" I asked, hoping against hope that he knew English. "...Ehhh... Hector...ehhh," he replied. "Where am I?" he asked shortly after. This question marked the beginning of a repetitious phenomenon. "Where am I?" he asked again before I answered him the first time. I found it normal to have asked the same question twice considering the elevated excitement and adrenaline a call can incur upon someone. "Where am I?" He asked a third time. "You're in the back of your house… do you know what happened Sir?" I responded to him the moment I heard a slight break in his anxious questioning. His original question continued and multiplied without waivering. "Where am I, where am I, where am I?" he constantly repeated resting on his backside in the dirt still.

By now, Jeff and I had concluded quickly that he was completely disoriented. The patient had concussed by way of the baseball bat, which made perfect logic, considering the crater he had in the posterior center of his head. "Where am I? Where am I?" His questioning continued as we secured him onto a backboard. —KSSHHH!!! "Dispatch, this is going to be a trauma alert, we'll be transporting to the nearest trauma facility". —KSSHHH!! "Will you need a helicopter or any additional units?" the female dispatcher inquired. —KSSHHH!! "No, that won't be necessary for now," I replied on my portable radio. Urgency bombarded the air. Jeff and I knew that our on scene time needed to be as fast as possible. After loading the patient onto our gurney, we hauled butt through the yard — this time the resistive terrain not being a factor. We flew toward the ambulance almost fast enough to have taken flight. We were comparable to an airplane on the runway during its initial take off.

Once inside the Ambo, my partner Jeff and I started two large-bore IV's, each of us on one arm, simultaneously. Running two fluid bags, one on each arm, we made a dire attempt to raise Hector's blood pressure because it was devastatingly low. Hector was well on his way into clinical shock had his blood pressure not been fixed! "Where am I? Where am I? Where am I?" Hector rattled off while in a cold sweat. His color was escaping his body due to the decreased blood flow. His pecan tan that resembled a rosy copper color began to diminish into a light khaki color. Completing our IVs prompted the control of his bleeding to provoke the cessation of exsanguination. Jeff applied a cling wrap viciously around Hector's head to plug up the relentless hole that constantly leaked a slow, oozing stream of blood. "I've got him all patched up with fluids running! Let's get out of here, now!" Jeff concluded.

It was my turn to drive us to the hospital while he maintained Hector in the back of the truck. I flipped on the emergency lights and sirens and applied light pressure to the gas pedal, looking to gradually gain speed as we rolled onward. Driving a big box such as an ambulance requires gradual, methodical driving, you can't whip it around like a go-kart or you're in for real trouble. Having only stopped a few times on the way at intersections, we arrived at the ER in no time. We were fortunate enough to only get held up by 2 out of 10 red lights. Red lights require emergency vehicles to stop too—we must make sure there's no knuckleheads flying through the intersection that may not have been aware of us or decided to simply avoid stopping. "We're pulling into the ER parking lot now, Jeff!" "Thanks bud," Jeff replied. "Where am I? Where am I? Where am I?" Hector's voice echoed from the back of the truck as I stepped down from the driver's Seat. I raced around to the rear door to dismount Hector. He sounded like a broken toy that had a defective talk button, the toys you're able to press and they speak a prerecorded sentence.

The trauma team was waiting for us with ready hands. Everyone stood in anticipation of our trauma alert patient. "He's got serious damage to his head…and evidently trauma to his brain," the trauma surgeon said, referring to the repetitive "Where am I?" from Hector. Jeff and I slid him over onto the hospital operation bed and two nurses closed the curtains after receiving a brief report on Hector. Later in the shift, a nurse who helped work on Hector confirmed that he had an open skull fracture. Whoever wailed on Hector with a baseball bat busted through *bone marrow*. It was likely that Hector would never be the same. Some say such is life. Others point to things such as karma. No matter how you place the blame or justify the reasoning, it doesn't change the end result. Hector is in my heart and in my prayers.

For God giveth to a man that is good in His sight wisdom, and knowledge, and joy. **Ecclesiastes 2:26**

#74

I'm Ready To Leave This Earth

Paramedic Pointer» *New drugs are constantly being developed. The commercialization process, however, takes years. The average time for a drug to be developed, tested and approved is about 9 years.*

Visiting nursing home after nursing home has gotten me acquainted with many elderly people. When I walk the halls of a nursing home, it forces me to ponder of where we will all end up in our old age. Just as I see the 88 year old woman in an assisted living facility, I also witness the 90 year old woman who still lives at home alone. Having witnessed these two instances on a frequent basis, my message to you as a healthcare provider and a dear friend is: *take care of yourself.* No one can *not* get old. Life is a race we all run and a person's age symbolizes how far along in the race that individual is. I say take care of yourself because though no one has found the fountain of youth, taking care of yourself will greatly better one's chances of living independently in old age. The last place on earth I would wish for somebody to end up is a nursing home. It's a babysitting facility for adults. I find it intriguing how humanity comes full circle at the end of one's years. We start out in diapers and we end up in diapers in our old age.

The second message I'd like to extend to the reader is: *find something meaningful to live for.* God wants believers to spread the gospel (good news).

Maybe you're not a believer and the gospel is irrelevant to you. You are still able to participate in loving your neighbor as yourself. Because whether you believe in God or not, exercising love is always appreciated.

A lady I met in a nursing home was loathing the absence of love — so much that she had attempted to kill herself. Our call shot to the computer screen, reading: *suicide attempt.* She was sitting in a wheelchair wearing a red cardigan and dress slacks. Her hair resembled cotton candy, only it was gray instead of pink and blue. A pregnant CNA, who appeared as if she was going to burst, escorted Jeff and I to the suicidal granny. "Here she is," the pregnant CNA told us as she pointed to a lone woman in a hallway. The patient had her head down in a shameful, depressing fashion. "We're your paramedics for today," I said as we walked into the granny's view. "What is your name dear?" I asked politely. She slowly picked her head up and said plainly, "Viola." "Very pretty name Ms. Viola... would you like to tell me why we are here today? Did you try to harm yourself?" "Yes," Viola said. "I took 20 nitroglycerin." Nitroglycerin is a drug that dilates one's blood vessels, causing a drop in blood pressure. A huge problem can arise in taking too many nitroglycerin tablets, and 20 is plenty enough to be labeled as too many.

What can happen is that the individual can very likely dump their blood pressure all the way to zero, leaving them with no pulse as well. After all, you can't have a pulse with no blood pressure to pump blood through your heart! "Why would you do such a thing to yourself Ms. Viola? What a terrible thing to do, there must be something seriously bothering you," I reasoned with her. "There is," she began. "My husband doesn't love me anymore. He put me in this terrible place and left me here... I don't even know why. He comes only once a week to visit me and when he does come, he doesn't stay long. I don't know why he won't let me come back home anyway, he won't let me leave this place and nobody cares... I'm ready to go home to the Lord!" she cried.

"Don't say that Ms. Viola, you must have kids and grandkids, dear!" "Yes I do, but I just feel like I have no reason to live anymore!" Viola began to whimper. The look she gave conveyed a sense of cluelessness as to what she was to do with herself. "I'm sorry that you feel this way, but what we can do is try and make you feel better. Jeff and I are nice guys and we'd like to see a smile on that face before dropping you off at the ER." She managed a soft, genuine smile. Viola's blood pressure wasn't nearly as low as we thought it'd be — indicative of her likely not having taken all that she said she did. Women are big fans of suicide by way of pills because it's less brutal and less physically traumatic. Whereas a man is more likely to jump off of a building or hang themselves.

The other thing about suicide is that many people, such as cases like Ms. Viola, will toil with suicide, but don't quite have the will to go through with it. Henry David Thoreau said, "Most men lead lives of quiet desperation and go to the grave with the song still in them." Live life to the fullest. Strive for greatness. Don't give up on your dream. And if things aren't panning out the way you would have them, keep pushing forward. Just keep going!

And lastly, be a warrior. Don't let life's problems and hang-ups push you out of your own existence. Committing suicide is conceding defeat. It's telling life that life was too much for you to deal with. But nothing is too great for you to deal with, especially with the power of God on your side.

And now, brethren, I commend you to God, unto the word of his grace, which is able to build you up, and to give you an inheritance among all them which are sanctified. **Acts 20:32**

#75

Epistaxis

Paramedic Pointer» When you have a nose bleed, pinch your nose and lean forward. Leaning backwards causes the blood to flow backwards, getting into the airway. Also, placing a handy ice pack on it will help control bleeding.

The medical terminology for a nosebleed is epistaxis. When I first began my pursuit of EMS at the age of 19, I couldn't understand the real purpose behind having so many interchangeable terms that meant the *same* thing — and I still don't, to be honest. Learning the medical term for everyday conditions we all see was like learning a second language, and in the hospitals it's a language your best interest is to be fluent in so you can function in that environment. But if you were to ask me, there's little to no reason for referring to one's kneecap as their *patella*. It's a kneecap for crying out loud, everyone knows that! Something tells me all of the fancy terminology was started by some smart Alec who wanted to feel like he was smarter than everyone and hence: the birth of medical terminology. I can just hear the person now rationalizing the idea in their mind, "Let's see… how can I one-up all of my buddies? Hmmm I know…I'll create a whole new language!" That's just my take on it. But honestly, nothing is so terrible once you get the hang of it, it just takes repetition.

A woman sat upright in a chair in front of a tailoring business. Four people surrounded her with hand towels as she leaned her head back as if she was stargazing in the middle of the afternoon. This woman looked to be about 70 years old, had pale white skin, and velvety white hair that was blood-tinged in some areas. Her shirt also had blotches of blood on the upper portion of her light blue top. Everyone helping her moved around her in a finicky panic, wanting something to do, but not being able to find anything more to help with. Walking up to the patient, I said, "Can anyone here tell me what exactly happened?" A woman looking to be about half of the patient's age stepped forward. "I'm her daughter…we were getting some outfits hemmed for her… when we walked out of the door to leave, my mom passed out and face planted on the sidewalk!" "How long was she unconscious for?" I asked. "Only about 10 or 12 seconds," she replied. "She woke back up and I got these people to help me put her into this chair," she said, pointing at the few other individuals on scene.

The 70-year-old patient's nose was bleeding profusely, it was deformed and crooked. It was evident to Jeff, myself and everyone else on the scene that she had broken it. Fainting is a result of sudden decrease in cerebral perfusion (blood flow through the brain). This time around we were lucky enough to have a witness that told us the culprit to the fall. There's a laundry list of why or how people fall, so it's up to paramedics to gather that back story the best we can. Having a witness helps out greatly and it allows us to choose the correct treatment modality in a fall patient, quicker. "Grab a c-collar for her, please Jeff," I requested. The patient needed her neck stabilized because of her head injury/trauma. Epistaxis can occur spontaneously or due to trauma, as in this tale.

A quick tip for stopping nosebleeds is to pinch the nostrils and lean forward. When you lean a child or anyone for that matter, backwards, it funnels blood into the airway and can cause choking. An additional helpful tip is to apply an ice pack over the bridge of the nose. This is done because blood vessels constrict when cold, reducing bleeding. That is the same reason ice packs are used for other injuries — reducing blood flow reduces swelling because that's what traumatic swelling is — blood pooling under the surface of the skin.

Applying our c-collar (cervical collar) to the woman brought about a great discomfort in doing so. The patient didn't appreciate the snug fit around her neck. Those collars are meant to help, but boy are they frequently unwanted! All we had to do next was obtain an initial set of vital signs (blood pressure, heart rate, breathing rate, etc.) and stand her up to pivot onto the gurney.

"Do you think we can stand you up hun?" I asked the sitting patient. "Mmmhmm…" she responded. Slowly rising to a standing position, she did a 180° turn to sit back down on the stretcher. Her turn was comparable to an ancient revolving door found in and *Indiana Jones* cave. "Here's couple seatbelts to keep you strapped in for the ride!" I said. "Jeff is a bit of a wild driver when he gets behind the wheel," I attempted to lighten the mood. The woman remained very calm, almost completely silent. No tears. No grimacing. No wailing. Not even a slight moan. Our patient handled her broken nose like a true All-Star.

I've seen grown men cry over an IV, so to see a grandma enduring this level of pain registered as impressive in my book. However, she didn't opt out of pain medication when offered. Jeff juiced her up with dilaudid to take the edge off. Falling to a young person may seem so trivial, but it gets much deeper than face value when a head injury is involved. Older people who are prescribed blood thinning medication can raise serious concerns for an internal bleed. Blood thinners increase bleeding. Also with the elderly, the brain reduces in size over the years, creating more empty space in the skull, which is a fixed vault. The elderly person's brain has a higher likelihood to smack against the skull when they fall and hit their head — known as a *subdural hematoma*. Our 70-year-old All-Star maintained consciousness throughout transport. With the help of a simple, but effective ice pack, her bleeding was stopped well before arrival to the ER. To Jeff and I's satisfaction, there was no internal bleeding going on inside her head once they performed a CT scan of her head. She only had to heal from her broken nose.

For I will be merciful to their unrighteousness, and their sins and their iniquities will I remember no more. **Hebrews 8:12**

#76

Dead For 3 Seconds

Paramedic Pointer» *Adenosine is an emergency medication used for patients experiencing fast heart rates. Adenosine slows conduction through the AV node (the heart's secondary pacemaker) in the heart. In other words, it "resets" your heart back to a normal rate. During the refractory period, patients experience a "flatline" heart rhythm for about 2-3 seconds!*

Never would I have guessed that the first words coming from a daughter's mouth when we showed up to help her dad would be, "Please don't take my father to the hospital!"— not from an *adult* anyway. But the 5'7" brunette was dead serious — to the point of tears. She stood in front of the Anna Maria Island mansion, drenched in tears of anxiety and pure fear. The mansion was tucked away in the corner pocket of the island. At the absolute northern tip of the island hid a cul-de-sac of multimillion dollar homes that could easily be missed without a GPS. The road the cul-de-sac of mansions lied on was hidden so well by the wild trees and monstrous plants, mixed with the cloak of shady darkness, that it's a wonder if anyone knows it exists.

"Please don't take my father to the hospital… the last time he went they kept him for four days! All he needs is *the shot*! Do you have *the shot*?! You guys…oh my gosh!" the middle-aged woman buried her face into her cupped hands and began bawling. I proceeded in taking out the stretcher. Sniffling, she started to speak, "I'm sorry... I'm just so stressed out right now with everything going on and it's just so much to deal with". *The shot* the daughter asked about happens to be a prehospital IV drug by the name of *Adenosine* that essentially resets one's heart. It's used in emergencies involving insanely fast heart rates. A normal heart rate for a healthy person is 60 bpm – 100 bpm, with the general exception being a professional athlete whose heart rate can tick as low as 40 bpm.

There are other unique individuals as well, but they are far and few in between. The cool feature regarding adenosine is that when given, your heart goes "flat line" for about two to three seconds — making you technically dead for a brief stint! "Where's the patient we're here for Miss?" I candidly asked the daughter standing in the driveway. Wiping her runny nose and leaky eyes, she told us, "My dad's upstairs lying down in his bed. He feels fine; he just needs the shot... that's all." "How peculiar", I thought to myself. "She surely must not know the seriousness of her father's condition if she's comfortable pushing for him to stay home without being assessed. Besides, leaving a patient home that we've given drugs is against our written protocol unless a doctor approves it; even then, it's a high risk decision. Jeff and I grabbed our medical equipment off of the cot and scurried up the plush staircase inside the mansion. Fixtures, lavish furniture and general high-quality decor occupied the interior of the costly home. This fella was living in style, to say the least.

Speed walking up the stairs and straight into the bedroom, we came face to face with a tanned gentleman, who appeared to be of Hispanic descent. His demeanor sent mixed signals, radiating an acute sense of irony. Here we were, rushing to an emergency, only to find a super relaxed gentleman, who appeared as if he didn't have the slightest care in the world. He lay comfortably in his satin, king-sized bed — surrounded by its royal purple sheets and pillows. Further, the man had a warm smile on his face.

"Oh wow, you guys made it here so fast! I'm so glad you were able to find my place, it's sort of tucked away back here," he exclaimed, his flamboyant personality shining through. "Anyways, I'm Soul... just to let you guys know, you won't need to transport me, this happened three weeks ago... paramedics came and gave me the shot; I got stuck in the hospital for four days and it was a total disaster. My doctor told me that if I gave him a buzz the next time my heart rate flew off the charts, he would approve of me getting the shot from you guys and staying home." Jeff shook his head in disappointment. "But what *you're* not understanding is that this particular drug stops your heart—I will literally be stopping your heart!"

Without hesitation, Soul responded with a big grin, "Yeah that's fine, I've already been through this." Realizing that he needed to be more specific about constrictions, Jeff replied, "I get it and I understand. What I need *you* to understand is that it's against my protocol to give you drugs — especially adenosine — and leave you home unsupervised afterwards. You could die!" "I know, I know" Soul said with his nonchalant grin. Jeff and I were paralyzed statues in hearing these words — we stood frozen in awe at the patient's carelessness on the matter. "This gentleman must absolutely loathe going to the hospital," I thought. "This just doesn't make any sense!" I continued to think. An awkward five seconds of uninterrupted silence passed by. Jeff and I almost had to pinch one another to see if we were dreaming because this was the most farfetched patient ever. Blinking fast repeatedly, as if he had woken out of a trance, Jeff shrugged his shoulders and grabbed his portable radio to key up the mic.

"Medic 16 has got a patient who wants treatment, but no transport, the patient is in a possibly fatal heart rhythm and has been explained the gravity of his current condition. What would you like us to do at this time?" —KSSSHHH! "Go ahead and treat the patient and revisit the decision to be transported with him after," the Doctor advised. "Okay we need an IV started and a bag of fluids hung. Also, 6 mg of adenosine needs to be drawn up," my partner Jeff announced. Three firemen had just joined the party, anxiously looking for somewhere to jump in. "If you guys (the firemen) want to get a bag of fluids going, Lorenzo and I will take care of the IV and adenosine administration." The entire time we hooked Soul up to our EKG cables (heart monitor) and acquired his vital signs, he sat there as if he was being waited on at a fancy restaurant. There was no fear in his eyes, which gave off both a vibe of bravery and eeriness.

"Have you got the adenosine drawn up yet?" Jeff asked me as he finished up his IV. "All ready to go!" I gave him an assuring response. "Hey…you may want to come over here and check the monitor out as Jeff gives him the ade-nosine… Soul is going to go flatline for a few seconds in just a minute… It's pretty wild," I spoke to the three firemen in a barely audible tone. Their inter-ests were peaked and they observed the cardiac monitor with uninterrupted focus. They didn't blink once. "Adenosine has been given!" Jeff announced. —"Holy cow!" The fireman standing right next to me whispered. It was like seeing a total solar eclipse for him. To see a person alive and actively propping themselves up in the midst of experiencing a flatline heartbeat is one of those weird instances you can only label as eccentric. It's the sort of thing that makes the hair on the back of your neck stand up. Soul continued to sit upright against his bed's headboard in complete comfort.

"Is my heart rate going down yet?" he inquired nonchalantly. Soul's heart rate had been as high as 232 bpm! Nothing safe about that. Not even remotely safe. At 232 bpm, one's heart rate is out of control. "It's going down all right," I responded as I observed the cardiac monitor. 232, 215, 200, 177, 143, 120… Soul's heart rate plummeted down drastically. His heart rate sustained at 115 bpm for a few moments. 115, 102, 93, 86, 80… Soul's heart rate continued to plunge. "Now we are within normal limits!" I said with great satisfaction. 80, 80, 80, 80… Etc. his heart rate leveled off once again, but this time maintaining a heart rate of 80 bpm consistently. Revisiting the decision to be transported or not, we consulted with Soul after about 10 minutes of monitoring him.

"You know guys, I really don't think that will be necessary so I'm going to opt out. Thanks anyway though, really," Soul said while nestled under his satin sheets. Shaking his head in disbelief once more, Jeff keyed up his radio mic again to consult with a doctor, this time stepping over into the far corner of the bedroom. As we waited for Jeff to finish up with his consult, Soul made small talk with the three firemen and I. "You guys see a lot of crazy stuff in this line of work…? What's it like having to work 24 hours in a row? You guys are so amazing…" He also offered us a glass of milk and some homemade cookies. We politely declined his hospitality, aiming only to keep things professional. Jeff walked back over to the foot of the king-sized bed, where the rest of us were standing in a bunch. "Never thought he'd go for it but our doctor says that he obviously prefers you to go to the ER with us, but we can't force you. He understands how adamant you are about staying home, so he instructed us to make certain that you know, as our patient, that you could very well *die*.

"Yes, I'm fully aware," Soul concurred. "Then with that being said and you understanding all the risks involved… sign here please," Jeff requested. Soul signed our electronic screen on our laptop and we cleaned up the mess we made. Medical supplies were strewn about all over his bed. "Have a good rest of the night," we told Soul. Soul smiled. "Call us back if you need us," I said. Because though he was doing well right at that moment, something told me that we'd be interfacing with this gentleman again. If not tonight, sometime soon.

And I will cleanse them from all their iniquity, whereby they have sinned against Me; and I will pardon all their iniquities, whereby they have sinned, and whereby they have transgressed against Me. **Jeremiah 33:8**

#77

Abdominal Atrocity

Paramedic Pointer» *Anytime we refer to a particular location of the body on a patient, for instance: the right arm, it is always the patient's right arm, not the right arm from our perspective.*

No matter how tough you may think you are or how hard you appear to be on the outside, abdominal pain can have one curled up in the fetal position, begging for mercy. There's a whole host of causes and underlying conditions behind abdominal pain. When abdominal pain arises, assigning a specific reason for it is comparable to picking a name out of a hat — it's more or less random.

Zone 16's call volume was running wild one blazing hot afternoon. This was no day to have your child walking around outside with no shoes on, or yourself for that matter. This call populated on our mobile screen right after Jeff and I had finished with a different call. We were tagged to handle this call because our previous patient refused transport, making us the closest unit — only two blocks away. Two minutes later we would find a black gentleman halfway falling out of the passenger seat of a teal Chevy Cavalier. I feared that he had a head injury because he was leaned down so far that his head was propping the rest of his body up. But it wasn't his head causing this awkward position he put himself in. He held his abdomen tightly with both hands, disregarding the absolute stress he was putting on his head.

Our patient had large, thick dreads so they may have padded his head a bit where it made contact with the pavement. The patient's body looked like he made an attempt to bail out of the front passenger seat, but only halfway successful. The teal Chevy Cavalier was parked in a resident driveway with the engine running. Out of the driver seat hopped a black female in a shower cap with pajamas on. She wore flip flops, revealing that her toenails were the same teal color as the Chevy Cavalier. Hands on her hips, she stood there, looking down at the black gentleman grasping his abdomen. Beginning to shake her head slowly in slight disappointment, she looked up at us and said, "I tried to take him up to the hospital, but he screamed as soon as I started the car… and that's when he opened his door and kind of fell out."

"Do you know what may be causing all this pain he's in?" I asked. "He just yelled 911… I think he does have a history of pancreatitis though," the woman exclaimed. Kneeling to get on the patient's level, I said, "Hello Sir, can you tell me your name?" No answer. Just the sound of straining. "I need to know your name Sir." More straining. Gritting his teeth, he said, " Demarcus." "Perfect, first we gotta get you off the ground and into my ambulance. Then we can look to treat this pain you're dealing with." Without any cue or warning, Demarcus took his back leg and thrusted himself out of the passenger car door. "AAHHHH!" he yelled. He coiled up into a tight ball and began to cry loud and hard.

Demarcus was as muscular as can be. His white tank top and sea of tattoos gave off the image of a heartless tough guy who had no conscience about anything. But his abdominal pain got the best of him today. Demarcus whimpered and whimpered some more. It was a really sad sight to see. Seeing a grown man cry so helplessly and shamelessly solidified the authenticity of his abdominal pain. There was no doubt in my mind that he was enduring great discomfort. And based off of his vitals, everything suggested great pain (I.E. a high heart rate and elevated blood pressure). Demarcus would not budge — he laid there in the driveway seeking comfort in the fetal position, which he did not find. Jeff and I had to pick him up and placed him on our stretcher.

During the lift he never uncoiled from his ball. It's almost as if we moved a human clam.

Tears poured down his face. Jeff and I moved quickly to juice him up with some much needed pain medication by the name of *Toradol*. Unlike our other selections of pain medication, Toradol isn't a narcotic. It's a lighter means of treating pain before we bring the big boys out. But if Toradol does the trick of alleviating the pain well enough, then our treatment stops there. Today was a day when Toradol palliated Demarcus's pain to the point of toleration. Demarcus improved enough to speak to us, which proved to be a 180° turn for the better. Pancreatitis is the inflammation of the pancreas, and there was no mistaking that Demarcus's pancreas was fully inflamed. However, there's nothing like a bit of prehospital management to get the body back on the right track. Just know that tough guy (or girl) or not, abdominal pain can have you begging for mercy.

For the Lord your God is gracious and merciful, and will not turn away His face from you, if ye return unto Him. ***2 Chronicles 30:9***

#78

Hypoxic Herman

Paramedic Pointer» *If you or someone you know is prescribed medication, be responsible enough to keep the prescription filled. Better to have it and not need it, than need it and not have it— especially when it comes to medicine that can save your life.*

Once a month or so, Jeff and I find ourselves running a respiratory call on the same gentleman by the name of Herman. It's not because Herman has *new* issues that constantly arise, it's because Herman chooses not to take care of himself properly. I'm not sure what you call someone who is fully aware of his asthma and kidney problems, but yet still chooses not to attend his scheduled kidney dialysis 3 to 5 times per week. I get it, 3 to 5 times per week, week after week is probably monotonous, tedious and quite frankly, no fun. But when it comes to your health, it just isn't in one's best interest to neglect their well-being. After all, who isn't willing to have their own back?— that's preposterous!

But in all actuality, reality says otherwise. And I'm a living witness to vouch for reality: chronic alcoholics, chronic smokers, 500 pound plus patients, hoarders residing in unspeakable living conditions… just to name a few. There's a pathetic amount of people perusing the world who don't give a crap about themselves, at least according to their actions.

Herman stood about 5'5" tall. He was a black gentleman with a round face. Shaped like an egg, Herman resembled a penguin in stature. Along with kidney complications, he also had a history of asthma, so each time Jeff and I responded to his house, Herman usually had on a nasal cannula. A nasal cannula is nothing more than oxygen tubing, equipped with prongs, to fit snugly inside one's nostrils. The crazy thing is, Herman answers the door every time doing his penguin waddle. The look on his face is as if what's going on with him is a surprise! "You knew you were getting low on your inhaler's medication," I want to say to him, but don't. "Herman, you knew your body would decline if you didn't show up for your kidney dialysis appointments!" — another thing I want to blurt out to him, but again, don't. You can't sit there and school your patients — especially in an emergency environment.

What we do is reinforce personal responsibilities in a professional manner by way of friendly reminders and suggestions. It's all a part of patient advocacy. Our job is to be the helping hands, not the disciplinary belt that delivers whippings. As usual, we sat Herman down on our cot and mixed up an albuterol/atrovent (breathing meds) cocktail in a nebulizer for Herman to breathe in. Albuterol and atrovent open up the airway, allowing a sufficient amount of air to flow into the lungs.

So eight minutes or so later, Herman's breathing returned to normal. His wheezes turned into normal breath sounds, clear on both sides, and his color came back fully. His kidneys, when not filtered via dialysis, contribute to numerous declines in his body's system. "Herman, you are aware that your kidneys are responsible for a great portion of filtering your body's waste, don't you?" I asked. "Yes Sir, I do," he answered. "I think it'd be best for you to stay on top of your treatments, could you agree?" "Yes, I'm going to start going regularly again," Herman replied. I believe that this particular emergency scared Herman enough to make a change. Because it has been quite some time now since I ran a call on him. The moral of this tale is: *take care of yourself.* According to the Bible, our bodies are a temple and I believe we should all treat it as such.

The wicked is driven away in his wickedness: but the righteous hath hope in his death. **Proverbs 14:32**

#79

Fainting On The Throne

Paramedic Pointer» *Paramedics learn their "ABCs", but it is a pneumonic, not just the mere alphabet. What we refer to when we mention using our ABCs is the order in which we typically assess our patients: A) Airway B) Breathing C) Circulation.*

Elvis Presley is said to have died on the toilet from a heart attack. What irony in his death: *The king died* on *the throne*, as some people refer to the toilet as, jokingly of course. What you might refer to as straining while on the commode is interchangeably referred to as performing a vagal maneuver in the prehospital setting. Essentially, vagal maneuvers reduce a person's heart rate. The only problem is that sometimes, usually an elderly person, can strain so hard that they reduce their heart rate to the point of passing out! Paramedics use vagal maneuvers (straining, or bearing down) in patients with insanely high heart rates. If we are unable to give vagal maneuvers a chance to improve a patient, it typically means that the patient is unconscious. This happened to be the precise case one early morning at a gentleman's house named Stanley.

From the time Jeff and I read the dispatch notes in our ambulance cab, we couldn't help but chuckle a little bit. The pre-arrival notes read, "Man slumped over on the commode." Our small chuckles quickly turned into uncomforting thoughts of a potential mess there could be in the patient's bathroom. Nobody likes operating in crappy conditions—I mean that literally. We'd soon find out, though, that our environmental preference didn't make a difference.

Answering the door was Stanley's wife. "Oh, I'm so glad you got here so fast… I thought that my husband was in the restroom unusually long… when I finally got off the couch to check on him… I found him unconscious… I was afraid he might be dead! He's still sitting on the toilet in the restroom just around the way there," Stanley's wife whimpered. Walking passed her vigorously, she told of how he'd been constipated recently. "He hasn't been able to move his bowels very well lately… I figured that's why he was in there for so long," she added.

There Stanley was — sitting atop the toilet seat with his head hanging down to the side. Stanley appeared to have had a rubber neck. Rushing in, Jeff and I shook Stanley, hoping that he had not lost his pulse. No answer. No waking. Feeling for a pulse, a faint throb could be detected at Stanley's neck. "He's not dead, so that's a good enough start," I said to Jeff. I quickly grinded my knuckles against his bony sternum in a second attempt to wake him up. No answer. No reaction. Not even a slight fidget. A sternal rub (the action I took with my knuckles) is a technique to intentionally discomfort patients so that they wake up.

Stanley's pants rested around his ankles. Peering between his legs, I saw toilet water, but no poop. Or as some say, there were no logs in the river. Putting Stanley's immediate history together led me to believe that he'd vagal maneuvered his way to unconsciousness. Everything added up to be just that. The wife saying he's been constipated. The fact that he was on the toilet (the place most people do any bearing down they are going to do). But the next clue we would find drove the nail in the coffin for evidence to show that Stanley was straining for relief. Slapping the blood pressure cuff on his upper arm, I took a quick blood pressure to gain a baseline. It was low. And his pulse was faint, yet rapid. Rise and fall of the chest was visible, signifying that our patient was breathing on his own. The piece of evidence to drive our conclusions of Stanley having beared down for too long showed itself quite presumptuously. I inserted my arms under Stanley's arms and lifted him off of the commode; he was to be pivoted onto our stretcher so that he could be wheeled out to the Ambo.

"Oh my gosh…" Jeff said with a look on his face that suggested he had seen a ghost. "What?" I said, intrigued with Jeff's stunned facial expression. "Look behind him…" Jeff answered. When I glanced behind Stanley, I saw a turd poking out of his buttocks — a gigantic one. Immediately, I sat him back down on the toilet to reevaluate the decision to sit him on the cot as he was. "What do you want to do about that?" I asked Jeff, referring to the massive piece of poop protruding from Stanley's backside. "Well we definitely don't want that on our stretcher… so I guess one of us will have to take some tissue and pull it out," Jeff concluded.

"Okay you lift him up again and you pull it out!" I encouraged him. Jeff stood there for a moment, trying to gather the courage to do the dirty deed at hand. All of a sudden we both heard a big plop in the toilet water. It sounded like a fish had jumped out of the ocean, making a small reentry splash back into the water. We both looked at each other, fighting the urge to burst into laughter. "Sounds like Stanley has been uncorked like a champagne bottle," Jeff exclaimed. Peering through Stanley's legs once more showed the brown plug that gave him such a hard time before we arrived.

Though the mass of feces had removed itself, Stanley remained in an unstable condition. His skin was pale, cool and moist. He was nothing short of lacking circulation in his body. Grabbing his underwear and pants, down around his ankles, I pulled them up as far as I could before uprooting him off the toilet a second time. Jeff and I placed him gently onto our cot and unzipped our blue medical bag to start an IV. "Go ahead and hang a liter of fluid because he's going to need every ounce of it," I told Jeff. Starting a large bore IV, we then let the fluids dump into Stanley's system. Before our transport was over, Stanley slowly came back around. "Who are you?!" he asked, as we came to a full stop in the parking lot of the hospital. "I'm a paramedic… we found you passed out in your bathroom!" "I passed out?" he questioned. "Yes, your wife was worried sick… but we figured you'd come back around because our fluid we gave you replenished the volume depletion your body experienced. "Wow… I didn't even realize I blacked out… thanks for the help," he said, staring off into the distance.

Stanley's color returned to him completely as we breezed passed the ER sliding doors. We had a delivery to make — Stanley. It was like a damaged good had been repaired before reaching its shipment location. Patched up. Mended. Restored. However you'd like to refer to it, Stanley was better now than he was when we found him. *Mission accomplished.*

*Blessed is the man that endureth temptation: for when he is tried, he shall receive the crown of life, which the Lord hath promised to them that love Him. **James 1:12***

#80

One Final Wish

Paramedic Pointer» *The 5 stages of the grieving process (in order) are: 1) Denial 2) Anger 3) Bargaining 4) Depression 5) Acceptance*

In my time spent as a paramedic, I've come across a sea of unexpected things. Smokers requesting a few more puffs on their cancer sticks before being transported to the ER — when they called for having *breathing difficulty*. The little old lady getting frisky with me or Jeff spontaneously without warning. Situations and comments that make you go, "Seriously??"

I'll tell you about a guy named Solomon who very well may be atop the list of unexpecteds. Nothing ceases to amaze me these days. But even still, over time, I am being desensitized slowly but surely. Each unique encounter chips away at what little innocence I have left. My tank for naivety has nearly run dry. Bone dry. I guess one could argue that that is the result of merely living in this world.

Our call happened to be smack dab in the middle of Williams Park. Williams Park is a breeding ground for homeless people. They sleep there, eat there, fight there and indulge in whatever other activities bums partake in — mainly sleep though. Williams Park is a place made for those who have more excuses than solutions. It's located in the heart of downtown Saint Petersburg,

Florida; lots of businesses, waterfronts and public buildings such as college and restaurants occupy that space. Walking by Williams Park one day trotted a man named Solomon — he had intolerable chest pain. Of course, Solomon wasn't walking still when we arrived at the scene. Solomon found a seat at the bus stop, where he waited to be evaluated.

"What's going on with you today Sir?" I asked the black gentleman wearing a formal vest and dress slacks. The outfit looked to be outdated, but clean by all means. "I was walking from the library... I was doing fine... and then my chest started bothering me real bad! I don't know if I can take it much longer... I feel like I'm dying," he said between breaths. Solomon sat there, slumped over, with both hands grasping his knees. "How old are you Sir?" "I'm 75 years old... Is there anything you can give me for this chest pain?" he inquired in between a heavy, drawn out breath. "Grab an oxygen mask out of the airway bag!" I urged Jeff. He quickly snatched one out of our green bag, hooked it up to the 02 tank and placed it on Solomon's face. "Breathe this in nice and deep, the best you can. And to answer your question— yes— we certainly do have something for your chest pain, Sir. But I need to take a quick picture of your heart before we do anything else."

"Okay just hurry, whatever you do!" "I know it's asking a lot right now, but try your best to hold still while our monitor takes a snapshot... it will really help minimize the disruption on our printout." 15 seconds passed by. Out came the printout of Solomon's heart rhythm and waveform. "He's not having a heart attack, but there certainly are imbalances and areas of concern. Get him loaded up!" I directed. Wires hung from Solomon's chest and limbs as we placed him onto the stretcher, which was right behind us on the sidewalk. I was happy to see that Jeff engaged the stretcher brake so that it wouldn't roll away on us. The only thing beyond the sidewalk we stood on was an extremely busy one-way street, filled with zooming cars. Heaven forbid our stretcher mistakenly rolled out into the tumultuous traffic!

In one fluid motion, Jeff and I picked up Solomon and placed him on the gurney. So much was going on in the midst of lifting the stretcher into the back of the truck. Bums paced by, trying to get a closer look at Solomon. A flock of birds made distracting noise just feet away. And of course, the rush of drivers speeding by, honking their horns at one another caused turbulence. "Focus," I ordered myself in my head. Safely putting Solomon in the rear of the truck, I tossed our medical bags inside and jumped in, closing the swinging rear doors swiftly behind me. Nitroglycerin sat just behind the see through cabinet that encased the medication with a sliding glass door. Taking the Nitro out, I gave Solomon a tablet to let dissolve under his tongue. Solomon's eyes closed, appearing to savor the medication tablet like it was candy. The next thing that came out of Solomon's mouth left me speechless. This man, who had endured chest pain, sweating, heart issues and breathing problems, all at once, voiced one important concern. Solomon, who found himself in a predicament with an outcome unbeknownst to him, had one last wish.

As he hung his head down, shaking it side to side with his eyes closed, Solomon said, "I only have one last wish I'd like to see come true before I die…" "What's that Solomon?" "… I want to have sex just one last time." He sat back against the stretcher and followed his statement with a long, drawn out sigh of satisfaction. He clearly felt as if he'd said enough with that statement. I'm not quite sure if Solomon knew that it takes a healthy enough heart to safely engage in such activity. Let alone, his being 75 a major deterring factor. I'm gonna leave his final wish alone at this point, because even today I remain perplexed at what was on Solomon's mind amid perhaps the most dangerous day of his life. With that, I'm going to take a long sigh myself and conclude with this final thought on the matter: "wow."

Fear not, little flock; for it is your Father's good pleasure to give you the kingdom. **Luke 12:32**

#81

A Comfortable Place Made For Dying

Paramedic Pointer» A hospice is a facility that provides care for the sick, namely the terminally ill.

A yellow sheet of paper rested on top of the nightstand beside the patient's bed with big bold letters—D-N-R. DNR stands for *do not resuscitate*, or in other words: "Don't you dare try to save this patient!" It's a piece of documentation put into place by either the patient themselves or someone close to them who make their medical decisions (usually a family member). DNR's are made with yellow paper due to that being mandated by the law. It makes it easier to find in a stack of documents, that's for sure. When a paramedic is handed a pile of papers regarding patient demographics and history, rather than thumbing through, looking for a DNR order, it's much more convenient to see a yellow sheet of paper because it *sticks out*. One of the emotionally low points for healthcare professionals is having to watch a patient decline before your eyes — to the point of death. And there's nothing much you can do about it but sort of help facilitate their comfort in dying. Give them some oxygen. Hold their hand. Reposition the pillow behind their head. But don't you dare pull out the defibrillators (shocking devices), needles or life-saving drugs.

And the shrewd legality of it all is that if you do go against the DNR order, you can be sued. That's right — you can be sued for saving someone's life when it's against their will. Which makes sense I guess, but it doesn't take away from the heartfelt moments that sloth by when all you can do is stand by and witness someone dying slowly until they croak.

Well that's what happened to a sweetheart named Cecilia. Jeff and I were summoned to respond to a facility built for dying people — a hospice. They offer a *comfortable way* to pass away, if there even is such a thing. And that was the irony in the call itself. Paramedics' jobs are to preserve life, so why call the resuscitation gurus for a person who is not to be resuscitated, right? This is where the order of things gets a little blurry because on a basic level, hospice patients can receive care, just not *advanced* life support or CPR.

Cecilia lay there, cute as a button, on her hospice bed. She currently had trouble breathing, and so her hospice facility wanted her to be seen by a physician. Her lips were purple from hypoxia (lack of oxygen) and her skin had a blue tint to it, also from oxygen deprivation. According to her paperwork, Cecilia was 68 years old. "Hello Miss Cecilia, I'm Lorenzo and this is my partner Jeff. We're going to slide you over from your bed to our stretcher so we can get you outta here, okay?" I said loudly as Jeff placed Cecilia on an oxygen mask.

No response. Cecilia didn't make a peep. She didn't even acknowledge my presence with her eyes. Without delay, we slid her over to our cot nice and smoothly. I had hoped that we would not be the ones to witness her slow motion decline to her utter ruin, selfishly enough. We made haste in pushing the stretcher down the long hallway to get her into our truck, which was parked under an awning just out front, beyond the facility's entrance doors. Looking down at Cecilia, her breathing efforts accelerated exponentially in a period of about 45 seconds. "Move faster, Jeff," I urged. But then I had the startling epiphany that moving faster, as with other patients, didn't increase Cecilia's survivability.

If today was her day to kick the bucket, that's all there was to it. Nothing Jeff, nor I did — outside of providing oxygen and general support — would produce a change in her inevitable outcome. A sense of impending doom suddenly sunk into my pores as I loaded her into the back of the ambulance. She began guppy breathing (like a guppy fish out of water), prompting Jeff and I to switch over to assistive ventilation with an oxygen reservoir that you squeeze to deliver artificial breaths. Our futile attempt to oxygenate Cecilia was the start of a sad case. Watching her go from pale, to blue, to purple, eroded the very fibers of my being. It dismantled my heart from the cavity of my chest wall, heaved it onto the ground and trampled it like a herd of mustangs dancing.

"Are you giving adequate breaths?!" I questioned Jeff. "Absolutely," he confidently responded. There were no other steps we could take at this point. I saw Cecilia's life force escape from her just seconds later. It's an indescribable event to see someone's energy escape from them, chilling really. There is no visual force that floats out of the person's body or transparent figure that ascends out of the individual's chest, but it's *there*. Nothing you can quite describe with the five senses but a sixth sense of some sort, activates, making one aware that someone has expired. Death. Misfortune at its best. Or, perhaps, the time one would sing "Oh happy day." My prayer is that on the day of your judgment, you have made sure prior that your trust is in the Lord, for he is your ultimate refuge and grace. Peace be with you, in Jesus name.

Trust in the Lord with all thine heart; and lean not unto thine own understanding. In all thy ways acknowledge Him, and He shall direct thy paths. **Proverbs 3:5-6**

#82

Night Club Chaos

Paramedic Pointer» *If you have ever experienced anaphylaxis (a severe allergic reaction with respiratory distress), you should obtain an Epipen®, which is an auto-injector prefilled with epinephrine. It provides instant relief from anaphylaxis when applied. This is where being proactive can save your life.*

Tonight was both a full moon and Halloween. Further, it was Friday, the perfect night to go experience a nightclub called *The Hall* in the local Tampa Bay area. Being Halloween, everyone stepped out to find some sort of mischief, whether innocent mischief or not. Every kind of person you could think of decorated the club's sidewalk, as they all waited in a line outside, formed against a brick wall. Our call came through as: *sick person*. Reading further down the ambulance dispatch screen revealed that there was a man down inside the nightclub. Instantly, Jeff and I jumped to conclusions, figuring that the issue at hand was either an assault or intoxication related. We all have heard the stories of the brutal bar fight or club outrage. Or about how someone overindulged on a random substance at the night club.

We got out of the ambulance and pulled our cot out, bringing every bag in preparation for the worst. What someone reports as a *man down* or *sick person* could actually mean *unconscious person* or *dead person*. Rummaging through the swarm of posers, wannabes, would-bes and copouts, Jeff and I dug deep enough through the dance floor to find our young gentleman, who appeared to be mulatto. He was face down with drool running down the corner of his mouth. He was out cold, as they say, with not a care in the world at this particular moment. First things first — we checked for a present pulse. Impetuous thumping of the base speakers jumbled up my focus slightly and jaded the detectability of a perfusing pulse — especially with the added barrier of a gloved hand. I managed to feel a pulse, nonetheless, and proceeded to turn our patient over onto his back. He reeked of alcohol, the scent seeped through his pores like heavy smoke through a vent. "He's had one too many, that's for sure!" I yelled to Jeff over the monstrously loud music. "Yeah, looks more like a few too many to me, man!" Jeff yelled back shaking his head.

We both positioned ourselves to lift the male patient onto our stretcher and vacate the building. "One… two… three… lift!" I shouted, raising the young male patient from the floor together with ease. "BLAAAHHH!!" — Out of nowhere, the patient began to vomit right in the center of the nightclub, spewing out nasty orange stomach contents. His vomit was projectile too, nearly spraying a nearby dancer dressed in a skimpy skirt. Though it managed to just miss the random female close by, the vomit ricocheted off of the ground and splashed my pant cuff just above my shoes. The patient's eyes were sealed shut while barfing his brains out, even to the point of flopping back against the stretcher's head. He appeared to be unmoved by what condition he was in, but the massive amount of alcohol would heed blame for that, hands down.

Jeff and I serpentined between a hectic mass of clubbers who twisted and gyrated to the beat of the music. Just as Jeff and I passed through the club's front entrance, our patient leaned over the side of the stretcher, almost hurling himself to the ground. He gagged, but no vomit followed. False alarm. It was only dry heaving. Jeff, who pulled the foot of the stretcher diligently with his back toward the patient, didn't realize what had happened. "Stop!" I yelled. Jeff halted. Turning around to see our patient hanging halfway off the cot, he kicked on the stretcher wheel brake before scurrying to the side of the cot to help me reposition him. Vomit, from our male patient's first upchuck rested on his shirt, beginning from his collar on down to his bellybutton. The stench invaded my nostrils and caused a bit of nausea in my body with each new whiff. One inhalation of any scent never hurt anybody, but recurrent invasion of the nostrils with an intolerable scent is when you begin to get overwhelmed.

Loading him into the unit, Jeff and I cleaned the mulatto patient up and instantly initiated an IV. An issue with drunk patients — especially when they have vomited a decent volume of stomach contents — is fluid replacement. IV fluid bags were put into place, being hung from the ambulance ceiling to deliver an ample amount of liquid into the patient's body. Moans and short spurts of gibberish came from our patient en route to the hospital. He even randomly reached out in front of himself and closed his fist as if he was grabbing something — all with his eyes still sealed shut. The gentleman, who looked to be 22, was completely wasted. Giving him the supportive care he needed, it was only a matter of time before he would return back to consciousness. But right now his altered mental status had him reduced to a sleeping baby having excitable dreams. So we did as any good set of parents would do and we carefully monitored the baby.

Trust in the Lord, and do good; so shalt thou dwell in the land, and verily thou shalt be fed. Delight thyself also in the Lord: and He shall give thee the desires of thine heart. Commit thy way unto the Lord; trust also in Him; and He shall bring it to pass.
Psalm 37:3 – 5

#83

The Treasure Chest

Paramedic Pointer» *A white, powdery appearance to the tongue is a sign of dehydration. Other signs include: poor skin turgor and light-colored mucus membranes (lower eye pockets and inside of bottom lip) instead of normal reddish color.*

Strip clubs have never been something that tickled my fancy. I've always loathed the thought of them from day one. Yes, as a man, I absolutely love an attractive woman — but not in the dynamic a strip joint presents women. Like any real man (emphasis on real), I enjoy genuine romance/love, true chemistry and monogamy. Not some showgirl auctioning herself off on a stage for a few dollars. Before this particular call, I had been inside a strip club all of one time and it was against my will — trust me. A buddy of mine's birthday brought all of the fellas together for a dude's night out on the town. We went out to eat, shot some pool and also went to a traditional dance club.

Around 1 o'clock that night, the birthday boy suggested that the night "Wouldn't be complete unless we all hit up a strip joint." We stood in a circle that night in a vacant parking lot. "Who's in?!" the birthday boy asked the five of us. Everyone raised their hands saying, "I'm in." Everyone except me.

I would have bid them all a good night but I didn't drive my own car that night, so I was somewhat at the mercy of the knucklehead I rode with. But I guess you can always get away from what you deplore if you try hard enough. I had an ex-girlfriend of three years who opted out of the relationship when the money got low and you'll never guess what profession she chose to run to (if you can even call it that). Stripping.

Did it tear me up inside? Absolutely. Did I contemplate violent, irrational actions to take as a means of revenge? You bet. But this all misses the mark in terms of forgiveness. Forgiveness, though it's not always easy, is what I believe in as a fellow Christian. If Jesus never died so that we all could be forgiven for our sins, we'd all be eternally damned. So choose forgiveness and I assure you that you will be blessed. God is our Father and awards blessings much like your earthly father giving you a pat on the back. It's a means of saying, "Good job son… I'm awfully proud of you." Betrayals in life happen, we have to learn to deal with it like civil adults. Remember how Peter betrayed Jesus by denying him three times before his crucifixion? God knows how you feel, no matter what you may be going through.

Friday night at approximately 3:15 AM, Jeff and I pulled up to a strip club by the name of *The Treasure Chest*. No one was outside initially when we pulled into the property. That is, of course, until a chubby white man was thrown out of the double entrance doors. He stumbled out onto the ground and face planted. His hair was in the style of a mullet and he wore a lime green tank top with khaki shorts. Soon following him out of the double entrance doors were two bald security guards dressed in all black suits. They wore black bluetooth devices in their ears as well that blinked a blue light every few seconds. Seeing as though our ambulance response was for an alleged assault, Jeff and I could gather that this gentleman was our patient. He looked like he had been roughed up pretty badly. We must've only caught the final licks he took from the bouncers in witnessing his violent exit from the club's entrance doors.

After lying on the ground for a second, the Caucasian male brushed off his kneecaps as he stood back up. He wobbled for a moment, his legs appearing to be one second away from buckling. The man appeared to be like one of those boxers who get spaghetti legs and collapse on the floor against their will after having taken a powerful uppercut to the head. He extended his arms out wide to maintain balance, just as a child extends his or her arms when walking along a balance beam. Looking around with eyes wide opened, he peered from left to right as if a stampede was coming around the corner, still barely able to maintain his footing.

"We'd better go get him before he falls down," I said to Jeff as we put our gloves on. "No doubt, this guy looks like he's fighting to stay on a tight rope or something!" Dismounting the ambulance cab, we rushed over to the wobbling man just outside the strip club. "What's your name sir?" I asked the patient. Shaking his wet mullet vigorously in confusion, he answered, "Uhhh Dan… my name is Dan". "What happened here tonight, Dan?" I asked. "OOWWWWW!!" Dan blurted, grabbing the back of his neck and rubbing it gently. Dan looked baffled as he tried to cope with the pain in his neck. Catching his bearings enough to speak again, Dan obnoxiously shouted, "They beat the F--- outta me…!! They beat the F--- outta me…! And I didn't do ANYTHING!"

"Okay but who?! Who did this to you? Who beat you up so bad Dan?!" I asked. "THEY BEAT THE F--- OUTTA ME MAN…! AND I DIDN'T DO ANYTHING!" Dan yelled again. His breath reeked of alcohol. He couldn't unglue his hand off of the back of his neck. Jeff sprinted to the Ambo to get a backboard and a C collar for Dan's neck. We performed a standing take-down— a procedure where you place the backboard up against a patient's back and glide them all the way to the ground, with the backboard against their back the entire time. Instead of having a patient simply lay down on the backboard, it allows them to do nothing, avoiding any unwanted spinal motion. Paramedics do not fool around with neck injuries because too many negative things can arise from a spinal injury. Dan jibber jabbered through the whole process of securing him to the backboard. It was as if he was completely oblivious to what was actually going on. His apparent alcohol consumption contributed to his spaced out nature, I'm sure.

Along with the fact that he was rattled from getting his butt whipped by the bouncer duo. A minute or two passed and Dan was now fully secured to the backboard. His head, now in a neck brace, was taped down as well. "THEY BEAT THE F--- OUTTA ME MAANNN…AND I DIDN'T DO ANYTHING!" he whined. Dan whined throughout the entire transition of getting from outside to inside the ambulance. While Jeff and I carried him to the stretcher he was whining. While we lifted him into the unit he whined. When I started the IV and gave him Toradol to take the edge off, Dan whined! All the way to the hospital, Dan's whimpering filled the truck. Arrival at the ER marked an elated release of endorphins throughout my body. Dan was one of the patients you were happy to help, but even happier to drop off. He spoke one sentence and now everyone at the hospital knew what happened without even asking. They didn't have to. Dan made it exceedingly clear that they had beaten the F out of him… and he didn't do *anything*.

I will not leave you comfortless: I will come to you. **John 14:18**

#84

Dying to Live

Paramedic Pointer» Don't bottle your emotions/feelings up. Over time, the pent up frustrations and aggravations you internalize will begin to eat you from the inside out. There's no shame in expressing disappointment or revealing your true feelings. Better to vent than to overheat and explode. Have your own back and give yourself a continual release. Paramedics must do this as well, not only due to the nature of the work, but because of the effects it has in our personal lives.

In my world of EMS calls there are constant cries for help in indirect ways. People acting out. People indulging in debauchery. People intentionally positioning themselves in the category of *failure to thrive,* which is the general failure to take care of oneself. Some people refer to these occurrences as individuals having abstract conditions. I refer to this as being *sorry.* There was no immediate medical condition for the call I'm getting ready to tell about, 911 got called for a simple lift assist — literally picking someone up who can do it themselves after they've fallen.

One could tell that the woman believed in God the moment one entered the residence due to the plethora of religious books, crosses and Jesus keepsakes on her walls. It's been said that you can tell what's on a person's mind by what they're reading and using that measure, she irrefutably had God on her brain! Making it back to her room revealed just why our female patient needed help getting up from the floor. She was easily 500 pounds. She had clearly fallen off of her bed because the mattress was tilted down towards the floor at an angle, halfway off of the bed frame. —KSSHHH! "Can I have an extra fire unit dispatched to this address…we're going to need an extra couple pairs of hands for our patient." The female Caucasian patient sat down on the bedroom floor with tears streaming down her plump cheeks.

"What's wrong Miss? You don't have to cry… my partner Jeff and I have come to help you," I empathized. "Are you in any pain?" I asked, noting that her tears looked more like tears of emotional dilemma or embarrassment. "Yes… yes as a matter of fact I am in pain… I've been in pain my entire life! I've got no family left, I'm lonely and I can't even leave the house because I'm so big!" she blurted out, followed by a shower of tears. "You can change your current predicament, Miss," I suggested. "No! I'm just ready to die and go to heaven so I can be happy again!" "Miss, you don't have to die in order to be happy again…let's try and be more positive!" I encouraged. We spent 10 minutes, or so, exchanging words until the team of firemen stepped in the bedroom ready to help lift her back into bed.

There's a sheet called a *patient mover* that has sturdy mesh material and handles on the outside for heavy lifting. Once we centered the 500 pound woman on the patient mover sheet (more like a tarp), we levitated her, so to speak, back onto her bed in a smooth fashion. No slippage, stumbling, or tripping occurred at all during that transition, which made me happy. Dropping a 500 pound patient, like any other patient, would cause harm — but multiplied by about four with this kind of patient.

The woman opted to stay home instead of go to the hospital, which in my opinion was a bad idea — but you can't kidnap someone, even if they obviously need an evaluation. She didn't injure herself from her fall out of bed. The reason why she needed to go get evaluated was because the bariatric woman had unsightly sores all over her body. "I don't want to be seen by anyone… I just want to die!" she cried. In conclusion, Jeff and I gave the woman uplifting words of encouragement and left her home, advising her to call us back the second she needed help and/or changed her mind about going to the ER to get evaluated. The reason I tell of people like this particular woman is because many of us, in one form or another, fail to thrive. We can't find a reason to get up in the morning, dreading life when life should be considered a gift from God. People like this are dying on the inside and often wish death upon themselves or contemplate committing suicide.

There is a God, who I call my father, who wants us all to live a life filled with happiness and love. This is a call for salvation, a gift of eternal life that can be granted to you right now if you accept Jesus Christ as your Lord and Savior. If you'd like to make the best decision you've ever made in your life then pray these words: *Dear God, I know that I'm and imperfect being. Please forgive me for all of my sins. I believe in your Son, Jesus Christ, and would like Him to come into my life so that I may walk more righteously, live out your will for my life and receive the gift of salvation. Open my eyes, show me truth and give me purpose Lord. Amen*

For the promise is unto you, and to your children, and to all that are afar off, even as many as the Lord our God shall call.
Acts 2:39

#85

A Mother's Worry

Paramedic Pointer» *Breastfeeding after delivery causes the uterus to contract, helping to stop postpartum bleeding. In addition, it also helps return the uterus back to its original size.*

Most mothers we respond to are petrified with anything involving their babies. A hiccup is reported as *choking* by terrified mothers. Any subtle temperature difference is automatically a fatal fever. Newborns, infants, and toddlers are extremely touchy subjects and as paramedics, we must treat these calls as such — even if absolutely nothing is wrong. Jeff and I responded to a one year old infant who swallowed a tiny bead. The house reminded me of a cabin. Everything on the outside and inside was wooden. Being located in a heavily wooded area gave the home a cabin in the woods effect.

One could tell that the family was enthralled with hunting. Each wall had a moose or deer head mounted firmly as trophies. Camouflage patterns were implemented in the little fixtures and props throughout the front living room. In the kitchen stood a male redneck with no shirt on and a brunette, Caucasian female holding an infant. Stepping towards us slowly was the shirt-less redneck with missing teeth. The bleach blonde hair on his chest and belly looked like it could glow in the dark. It was golden and puffy. Scratching his belly, the Caucasian man said, "We are really worried… this is my sister and nephew," he exclaimed, pointing towards the brunette holding the crying baby. "My nephew swallowed a tiny hair bead and we're not sure what to do… his eyes had a red tint to them when he began crying."

— "My baby was crying tears of blood… my baby was crying tears of blood!" the woman cried. "He wasn't crying tears of b… — "My baby was crying tears of blood!" the woman interrupted the uncle, who tried to say something. "What exactly did the tears look like…? I mean, are you sure it was blood that you saw?" I said as I pressed the stethoscope against the infant's back to listen for lung sounds. "Rachel… calm down… let me talk…" the shirtless man pleaded as he shot her a cautious glance. She nodded in acceptance of his request. "Okay… there *looked* to be a red tint in one of the tears that ran down my nephew's cheeks… but it very well could have been because his eyes were red in general after he cried for a bit. But it did not look like tears of *blood*!" the man said confidently. The mother concurred, in approval of what he told Jeff and I.

We continued our assessment (listening to breath sounds, evaluating the infant's eyes, mouth and more). Everything came back with no real concerns. "The number one concern we have for your son is the patency of his airway, having swallowed a small object. Due to your baby crying, he clearly has an open airway. His eyes do have a red tint to them, yes, but that's not abnormal for a crying baby. We would gladly take your son on down to the hospital if you'd like, but what's gonna happen is your son will poop out that hair bead. It's not lodged in his airway," I concluded. "You don't think he needs to be seen?" she asked in a worried tone. "No, if you'd like us to take him on down, we'd be glad to, but we don't feel you have anything to worry about." "Okay… I'll get him checked out at the doctor then," she said softly. "Thank you for helping us… I was worried sick."

To the loving mothers out there, remember one thing — if anything — about this tale when you suspect that your little nugget is choking… a crying baby is a good baby in terms of airway concerns! If the baby is crying, a foreign object isn't blocking the passage for airflow. Think about it, have you ever been able to verbally make cries in the midst of choking? Take care. And remember: *look twice at things you have concerns about.* Wouldn't want to mistake a red tint to the eyes as tears of blood!

Even a child is known by his doings, whether his work be pure, and whether it be right. **Proverbs 20:11**

#86

Hardworking Breadwinner

Paramedic Pointer» *"Burning the candle on both ends" can be necessary, at times, but don't overdo it. Give yourself adequate time to rest and replenish lost nutrients when working hard or exerting yourself in general. If you can't make the decision to give your body a break when it needs one, eventually your body will make that decision for you!*

Men have the tendency to bear ridiculous amounts of pressure. Many men take on the responsibility of working long hours to provide for their stay at home wife and children. Women bear great responsibilities too, but this is a story of how one young family man took on more than he could handle. Or as some say: "He bit off more than he could chew."

Jeff and I responded to an apartment complex that had dirt lawns instead of grass lawns. The sidewalk ran parallel to the row of apartment units about 30 feet from the doors. There was a dirt lawn, sidewalk, and then more dirt out by the mailboxes, until the dirt met the concrete road.

Walking into the front door, which was propped open halfway already, I saw a young white male — about 28 years old, sitting leaned back on the couch next to a blonde female who looked to be about 25 or so. He was sweating profusely — the blonde female appeared to be overwhelmed with anxiety, nestled snugly under her husband's arm. "What's going on today, Sir?" I asked candidly. "I'm not exactly sure, to be honest with you," he answered. "… I just feel weak all over… I had to cut my shift short tonight and come home," he said, beginning to breathe more heavily. "Understandable…what do you do for a living?" I asked him. "I'm a trucker… I work long hours… 16 hour shifts… sleep eight hours, pop up and do it again… one thing I can say is that my heart feels like it's beating fast! This has happened to me once before when I was at a rest stop… I fell out of the driver seat and had to army crawl all the way to the bathroom!" "Were you ever seen by any medical professionals about why you got so weak all of a sudden?" I inquired.

Looking to be embarrassed, he focused his eyes on the ground and said, "Umm no." "Okay so we've really got no insight on what's causing this sudden onset of weakness besides you being a workaholic," I concluded as Jeff hooked up our monitor wires. "Wow! Your heart rate *is* beating really fast! What were you doing at work? Anything strenuous?" I quickly questioned. "Nope, just driving long hours, pretty much. I've drank five energy drinks though… they're what keep me going… I count on those bad boys!" While looking at the male patient, I'm thinking, "Aha… no wonder… there *is* a potential culprit to these issues he's experiencing at such a young age." Letting my thoughts marinate for a few seconds, I then said, "Well that's a problem in it of itself. Your consumption of those energy drinks seems to be tearing your body up. Drinking five and six of those energy drinks per day wears on the body over time," I exclaimed.

"Yeah I know, it's just that I've got a family to take care of," he said, as he shook his head. "Well your body isn't agreeing with those energy drinks as you can see, my man," I told him. Jeff hooked up the cardiac cables to the gentleman's chest to take a picture of his heart (12 lead EKG). As the printer's paper rolled out of the cardiac monitor, Jeff said, "It's looking pretty clean, just as we'd expect a 28-year-old's heart to look." Our patient let out a sigh of relief. "But your heart rate is still fast… that's a real concern for us, Sir," Jeff exclaimed. "Why don't you take a trip on down to the hospital with us tonight?" I chimed back in. "Sound like a plan?" "Yes, that's fine… whatever you guys feel I should do." The young family man kissed his wife and baby daughter following Jeff's completion of his IV.

"Your enzymes may be imbalanced or something… but the ER will find that out when they draw blood. You've gotta take a little bit better care of yourself, my man… you don't want to overload your system like you've been doing," I added. The patient looked completely fried from working himself to death. He proved to be stable during the transport to the hospital; he likely needed fluids such as water to flush out his system. Sort of like replenishing one's self with water after a night of heavy booze drinking. My message to the reader via this true tale is *don't overwork yourself.* Maybe you've got young kids and a spouse to look out for, but just remember that you can't be of any help if you get hospitalized. Bills don't stop and mouths don't stop getting hungry — I get it. But that doesn't mean we all can't be wiser, plan more strategically and implement time management more effectively; not to mention, monitor the things we consume with our bodies.

He shall call upon Me, and I will answer him: I will be with him in trouble; I will deliver him, and honor him. **Psalm 91:15**

#87

Paranoid Patrick

Paramedic Pointer» *Both recreational and medicinal drugs may induce side effects or what is called an adverse reaction. The difference is that side effects are expected, whereas an adverse reaction is a unique response to the drug.*

Beware of what recreational substances you snort, ingest, shoot up, smoke, huff, etc. — not that you should be doing that sort of thing anyhow. First, I'm going to give you biblical advice since it's my duty as a believer in Christ, and then I'm gonna tell you of a particular recreational drug call that went south.

The Bible speaks on the subject of *debauchery*, which means the excessive partaking in of unnecessary pleasures. God doesn't want us to partake in such pleasures as getting drunk and high all the time because it leaves us *stagnant*. Also, he sees our bodies as a holy temple, one that should be taken care of with great responsibility. Being high or drunk may feel good, yes, but it impairs our judgment, especially when we indulge in it excessively.

Patrick was a 30-year-old mulatto man who Jeff and I were fortunate enough to meet while having to cover a call for zone 12 — the zone next to our home district — zone 16. The apartment complex Patrick was located in had an exterior made of red brick. It was called *Carlton Arms*. Patrick lived on the second floor, where we found him sitting on the edge of his queen sized bed. He had his legs crossed like a classy gentleman, appearing to be contemplating the wonders of the world. He looked so relaxed too, as if nothing under the sun could faze him. Before we made it all the way to Patrick's bedroom, we came upon a black female pacing back and forth in the kitchen with a cell phone glued to her ear. Worry took over her — I could practically hear her heart beating from 5 feet away.

"Something's wrong with him — he's not acting normally! I'm his girlfriend Stephanie by the way… I've been here for three hours or so." "When did he start acting out of character…? What were you two doing when the change in behavior occurred?" Stephanie stared at me for a moment, trying to decide whether to give me the honest truth or not. She attempted to read my face as if to decode whether I would run and tell the cops or not like a snitch. Seeing that she couldn't make up her mind, I interjected. "Stephanie… if you're concerned about me having a problem with any drugs, let me just say that we are *not* the police. We are all medical professionals here," I assured her, pointing at Jeff and the three firemen on scene with us. "We don't care about the fact of whether what you all were doing was legal or not… we want to know this information because of the importance it has concerning our patient's health," I exclaimed.

Following my short heart to heart explanation, Stephanie gained the confidence in us to give us the straight skinny. "We were drinking wine, smoking weed, and ate a few shrooms. We wanted to take a trip… mine was fine, but his wasn't so good. He started freaking out on me and told me to leave. That's when I came into the kitchen and called you guys." "Thank you so much Stephanie… you've really helped us out a lot… a big portion of these patient outcomes relies heavily on knowing what happened, medical history and things of that nature. It helps us decide how to go about treating the current issue." Giving her a warmhearted smile, I turned — along with the rest of my crew — down the hallway to evaluate Patrick.

There he was, as far on the edge of his bed as he could possibly be without scooting all the way off. Atop his nightstand sat a collection of empty alcohol bottles. Incense burned elegantly on his clothing dresser. We all could smell a potent scent of marijuana coming from somewhere, but couldn't place our eyes on it. Patrick bounced his leg — the top leg that crossed over his knee. He looked so serene, much like the general environment of his bedroom. He was so relaxed that he hadn't even noticed the five of us barge in with medical equipment. One couldn't tell if Patrick expected our arrival or just got lost so deeply in a trance that he became frozen in amazement. "Hey Patrick…" Jeff said, breaking the eerie silence in the bedroom. No answer. Patrick didn't even break his motion of leg bouncing.

We all moved a few steps closer to him, expecting that he would then notice our presence. —Still no reaction or awareness to the five of us. "This is mighty strange," I thought to myself. A fireman stepped forward and shook Patrick's shoulders, "Hey brother, can you hear me… we are EMS… we've come to see what's going on with you," the fireman spoke directly into his ear. As the fireman stood back up straight from leaning into Patrick's ear, Patrick turned his head slowly and calmly asked in a gentle tone, "Who are you?"

Before the fireman could answer, Patrick asked him again, this time with a wee bit more urgency. "We are EMS… we came because your girlfriend called 911… she said that she was concerned about you because of the way you were behaving… 'Out of your norm' is how she described it… — "Wait," Patrick interrupted. "Who are *you*?" he said, focusing on Jeff. "And you guys… who *are* you people?! Who are you people and why are you here?!" Patrick screamed in a fit of rage. A moment of awkward silence lapsed — we all were caught off guard by the seemingly bipolar episode Patrick was having. Just as quickly as Patrick became loud and obnoxious, he became instantly forlorn. Looking to be innocuous, Patrick turned red hot and then back to lukewarm all in a matter of five seconds or so.

Falling down face first into his pillow, Patrick threw his hand up as if to stop us from coming any closer to him. "Please don't hurt me! Please don't hurt me guys! I'm sorry! I'm so sorry!" he whimpered with his face buried in the pillow. Me and the EMS gang exchanged baffled looks at one another. Attempting to proceed with an evaluation, I placed a hand on Patrick's shoulder. "It's okay buddy… we are here to help. We need you to sit up so we can…" — "DON'T TOUCH ME… AHHHH! —NO! WAIT! I'M SORRY!" he whimpered. "OH GODD WHAT'S HAPPENING TO MEEE!?" Patrick cried. His emotions changed colors like a chameleon and the rate his mood changed was uncanny. No one knew what to expect from this guy. "I don't know what's happening to me, I just… I'm just so scared… so scared," he exclaimed. "Why don't we sit you up and take some vital signs before we do anything else… fair enough?" "Yes sir," Patrick agreed.

It was an interesting feeling being called "Sir" by someone who was so close in age to me, yet older nonetheless. Being 25 and called Sir very sub-missively by a 30-year-old just kind of felt out of order. Vital signs proved to be unremarkable and his blood pressure came back within normal limits. Pulse rate, breathing rate and blood sugar all fell within normal range as well. Patrick's skin was sweaty though— abnormally sweaty. And his hands were so sweaty that there wasn't a chance that he'd be able to grasp anything if he tried. Paranoia submerged Patrick like he was locked in a fish tank. He had experienced a bad trip with the drugs and it resulted in a panic attack.

Anxiety sweeps people off their feet so bad that some have to go and get prescription benzodiazepines such as *Valium* to manage it. Our ride to the hospital was relatively serene. Patrick revealed that he's a true to life wine drinker, consuming easily 7 cups of wine per day. He told of how he was an orphan for many years until his adopted parents began taking care of him. I empathized with him, telling him how we've all been dealt different hands, so to speak, but how God gives each of us particular gifts to make do with what we've got. It's going to sound cliché but it's just so true: *when life hands you lemons, you've got to have the willpower to strive forward and make lemonade!*

Patrick became very fidgety when we arrived at the hospital. His shaky hands frantically grabbed at the stretcher seatbelts to unbuckle them. "Oh no… you guys aren't going to take me into the ER on this thing are you?!" Patrick asked as Jeff and I unloaded him out of the rear ambulance doors. "What are you doing — don't unbuckle yourself Patrick… if you fall off the stretcher, then a whole host of liability issues arise, so please… stay put my man," I said calmly with my hand on his wrist. Patrick loosened his grip on the seatbelt buckle and attempted to relax. "I just don't want people looking at me, I'm a complete wreck and it's embarrassing!" he began to tear up again. "You've got nothing to worry about Pat," I assured him. "I won't leave your side buddy," I added. "You won't?" he asked, looking up at me with puppy dog eyes. "Nope" I replied. "Okay," he said.

As soon as we got in the center of the ER, where patient registration takes place, Patrick began to freak out again, starting with a few tears cascading down his tanned cheeks. "OH MY GAWDD…WHY IS EVERYONE LOOKING AT MEE!? This is so embarrassing… I'm so scared!" Taking a moment to peer around the facility, I saw for myself that no one was paying any attention to Patrick at all. It was all in his paranoid mind. Patrick had become delusional, as if paranoia wasn't enough. "Don't leave me… please don't leave me… stay right here with me…" Patrick urged me. He was scared out of his mind — like a child who had just seen the boogie man. I promised not to leave his side. Soon after our verbal exchange, an attractive nurse came to take report from me, regarding Patrick. Once we transferred Patrick over to the hospital bed, he passed out before Jeff and I even announced availability for the next call.

The fear of the Lord prolongeth days: but the years of the wicked shall be shortened. **Proverbs 10:27**

#88

Falsified Falsetto

Paramedic Pointer» *Paramedics are investigators when it comes to patients. A pneumonic we use to narrow down the immediate problem, when asking questions, is S.A.M.P.L.E. This stands for: signs and symptoms, allergies, medications, past pertinent history, last oral intake and events leading up to the current predicament— It's a way of extracting necessary details for our medical care.*

The *falsified falsetto* is a false alarm, simply put. It's the boy who cried wolf. —The person who stubbed their toe. —The bum who wants a place to sleep at night, and since a hospital looks a lot like a hotel in comparison to sleeping under the highway, a falsified condition or injury is made up to get a warm bed and a meal. Another form of a falsified falsetto is when a civilian drives by someone and decides to report for that person that they need an ambulance. In EMS, we refer to those drive-by callers as *cell phone heroes*. A cell phone hero won't get out of their car to check if a homeless person is just sleeping rather than dead, they'll just call and state that "someone might be dead on the public bench."

But you have to be mindful of the cell phone heroes who pose as anonymous Good Samaritans, because sometimes the motive is to simply remove a bum from a lot or public bench because it bothers them. Like an eyesore.

I'll tell you about a so-called Good Samaritan who recognized a sight that made his eyes sore, all right. What he saw sent him into a panic, and he had to do something without getting too involved. So, as you may imagine, he opted to phone the paramedics. It was 6 o'clock in the evening — a call populated on our ambulance computer screen stating that someone was experiencing seizures in the parking lot of a car dealership. The dealership general manager was the caller. We cruised slowly past the car dealership searching for our alleged seizure patient. There simply wasn't enough space to fit the huge ambulance in that tiny parking lot, so we did one Slo-Mo drive by, busted a U-turn and inched passed the parking lot again.

Out came an Italian man, middle-aged, wearing a bright yellow shirt and about three bottles of hair gel in his head. His hair was slicked and shiny, full of shimmer. He stood out by the street curb with his hands on his hips. A look of grave concern masked his face. Hopping out of the ambulance, Jeff asked, "Where's the patient?" Looking down at the ground briefly in disappointment, he shook his head and said, "The old lady is probably across the street by now…" Though he seemed to be greatly disappointed, he also appeared to be traumatized beyond measure. "What was going on with this guy?" I thought. People react differently when they witness a seizure; I noted that as a potential explanation for these mixed signals I was picking up from the dealership manager. But there was a problem with that being the potential case. He stated that the woman was probably across the street, which would mean that she's up and moving.

People who've experienced a seizure don't typically get up and move from here to there afterwards. Not immediately anyway. Registering this in my mind, I asked, "So why did she need 911?" Or in other words, "Why did *you* decide to call 911, Mr. Manager?" "Uhh…" the general manager began. "The woman… ahh" he sighed. —"Come with me and I'll just show you," he said. He walked over in between two cars on the lot and pointed. One could smell it before seeing it, if that means anything to the reader. There on the ground, before us, lied a pile of human feces. Jeff and I stood in complete awe of the disgusting sight before us. It smelled like, well, it smelled like exactly what it was. A pile of crap!

Peering across the street, I spotted an old woman who looked to be about 70 years old, hunched over. She staggered about with the help of her geriatric walker. "There she is," I said aloud, pointing across the busy street. She was staggering about — yes — but make no mistake that she was moving along quite nicely, moving forward with great intention and purpose. She seemed to be trying to escape; after all, she was fully aware that she had dropped a load of human defecation in between the two dealership cars, that's for certain.

Cutting our conversation short with the general manager, Jeff and I excused ourselves and made our way across the busy road to catch up with the old woman. "What do you want!?" the old lady snarled. "We just came to make sure you're okay, that's all." "I'm fine!" she answered with an ill-tempered tone before turning her back to us and stumbling forward. The toe of her shoes drug against the sidewalk's pavement. Her legs weren't even in length, so she walked with an exaggerated limp. "Where are you going?" Jeff asked. At this point we stopped trailing her heels. The old, hunched over woman turned around with a scrunched up face and said, "I'm going *this* way!" and proceeded to turn back around slowly and keep pacing onward. Jeff sighed. "Let's just let her go... there's no sense in continuing to chase her... she's clearly okay." "Yeah, no kidding," I agreed. I documented my report stating, "Patient fled the scene." We just don't have the time to chase down folks who don't want help. Or even need it, for that matter.

For by Me thy days shall be multiplied, and the years of thy life shall be increased. **Proverbs 9:11**

#89

I Dropped My Breath...Help Me Catch It!

Paramedic Pointer» *The primary function of the respiratory system is to exchange oxygen with carbon dioxide.*

Respiratory arrest is a very critical event that can take place in a patient. It's when a person stops breathing *altogether*. Unlike cardiac arrest (no breathing, no pulse), there may be a pulse in a patient who is completely absent of any breathing. Respiratory arrest is highly volatile, nonetheless, as you may already imagine, especially when the cells in one's brain begin to die off, one by one, after about 4 to 6 minutes of receiving no oxygen.

Mr. Crutchfield knows what it means to experience a bout of respiratory arrest — and live through it — with some help of course. And that's where my partner Jeff and I came in. Having an average day in zone 16, we were discussing football over lunch, when the emergency tones rang. "You better slurp down the rest of that chili unless you plan on leaving it here… it's time to rock!" Jeff exclaimed as he scooted out from beneath the kitchen table. Our call notes stated that an 86-year-old male had breathing difficulty. Little did we know that it'd not only be breathing difficulty, but the total absence thereof! We pulled up to an assisted living facility called *Westminster Shores* — a nearby place in zone 16 — where elderly patients frequently got transported from. Mr. Crutchfield lay in his bed with a nasal cannula resting in his nose, which delivered supplemental oxygen.

"Mr. Crutchfield has a history of asthma, chronic obstructive pulmonary disease and congestive heart failure. He's been dealing with them all for quite some time now and he's been under close monitoring," a nurse stated. Jeff hooked up the oxygen saturation probe (a finger probe to monitor how well a person is breathing) on to Mr. Crutchfield. I attached the cardiac cables to our patient simultaneously. "His 02 reading is dangerously low!" Jeff said aloud. "Here's the nonrebreather (02 mask)! Put it on him!" I replied to Jeff.

After placing Mr. Crutchfield on high flow 02, his oxygen reading only increased a couple of points — still too low to support life. "Where's the intubation kit?!" I said frantically. Jeff hurled the blue intubation bag at me. Mr. Crutchfield's breathing had decreased considerably, to the point of being unconscious. But he still breathed, in a labored fashion, slowly declining every few seconds. In the meantime, Jeff delivered assistive breaths to the patient as I prepared to intubate Mr. Crutchfield. Intubation, for the reader who does not know, is the process of placing a breathing tube down a patient's trachea (windpipe) to deliver oxygen into one's lungs. "Okay Jeff, in about three seconds I'm going to go for it," I said, referring to an attempt at intubation.

Glancing down at Mr. Crutchfield, it had become apparent that all breathing was completely from Jeff's manual squeezes of an oxygen reservoir that we paramedics call a *bag valve mask*. Mr. Crutchfield had acquired a purple tint to his skin due to the oxygen deprivation. "He definitely went into respiratory arrest! It's a good thing we got here when we did!" Jeff stated. "All right Jeff… I'm ready!" I declared while hovering over our patient's head, holding my tube and laryngoscope blade. Jeff moved out of the way and I proceeded to intubate Mr. Crutchfield after locating the anatomical landmarks that are so crucial for success. There are a few landmarks one must identify as reference points, but there is no ignoring the vocal cords — two white slivers that one must pass the oxygen tube through. Paramedics refer to the white vocal cords as the *pearly gates*.

"I see the cords… aaannnd… —there we are!" I celebrated. "The tube is in! Help me get him slid over to the stretcher, Jeff!" I said. A critical part of Mr. Crutchfield's survivability had now been accomplished — his airway was under our control. Jeff and I wheeled Mr. Crutchfield out of *Westminster*

Shores as fast as we could without tipping the stretcher over as we bent the corners. The patient's color slowly regained, little by little, following each breath delivered. Jeff's squeezing of the bag valve mask replenished Mr. Crutchfield's overall appearance en route to the ER, which brought satisfaction to us both.

A paramedic's goal is to drop off a patient looking better than they did when picking the patient up. Today our goal was accomplished. And further, Jeff and I later found that Mr. Crutchfield returned to a fully functional state after receiving critical care from the hospital. As your paramedic, spiritual advocate and friend, I ask that you stay away from unhealthy habits such as smoking. I know, it may sound cheesy and cliché, but this is how respiratory diseases such as emphysema begin! God wants to see you do big things — it'd be a pity to cut your blessings short by making silly decisions.

For whosoever shall do the will of my Father which is in heaven, the same is my brother, and sister, and mother. **Matthew 12:50**

#90

Lost Ones

Paramedic Pointer» A miscarriage is the spontaneous loss of a woman's pregnancy before the 20th week. Miscarriages often occur because the fetus isn't developing normally. Unfortunately, the miscarriage process can't be reversed once it has started.

In the wee hours of the morning is when zone 16 finally gives Jeff and I a break from running our butts off — the majority of the time anyway. The hours of 3 AM to 6 AM seem to be the golden hours, as I call them. No matter what day it is, it seems to be the window the night crawlers have just fallen asleep and the early risers have not yet awoken. But the harsh reality is that emergencies never sleep, despite the fact that a paramedic works 12 and 24 hour shifts.

3:30 AM marked the final call of the shift for Jeff and I when the dispatcher tones sounded off. Those invasive alarms catapulted my partner Jeff and I out of bed to don our reflective jumpsuits we wear during nighttime. "Medic 16... abdominal pain/obstetrics related," the electronic female voice disclosed. "It would be just our luck to deliver a baby as our final call for the shift," Jeff said, shaking his head. Revving up the truck, we filled the ambulance bay with smoke before taking off. "We're going to have to get that checked out before it's too late... did you see that cloud of white smoke back there?" Jeff asked as we pulled into an empty street in front of the medic station. "Yes, did you break the truck again?" I said jokingly. Jeff shot me a side eye. Virtually no cars were on the road this time of morning, relinquishing the need to use any sirens. Instead, we just kept the flickering red lights flashing for visibility purposes. No need to part an ocean of cars like Moses did the Red Sea — not on this call.

Arriving to a dark condominium lot, a large Caucasian woman came into view. She leaned over in pain, resting on the trunk of a white Ford focus. Next to her stood a Caucasian male providing moral support with a gentle hand on her hip. The Caucasian man was only half the normal height of a person — he had nubs for legs. It looked as if he were kneeling down on both knees, but there were no flesh below his thighs. "It's okay honey, it's okay… everything will be all right," the man said. Walking up to the couple, I inquired, "What's going on with her?" The 3 ½ foot man replied, "She's having belly pain… she thinks she might be having a miscarriage!" he advised.

—"GIVE ME SOME MEDICINE FOR THIS PAIN! IT'S THE WORST THING I'VE EVER FELT!" the woman yelled. "How many weeks pregnant are you?" I quickly asserted. "18!" the woman grimaced in pain. Jeff swung the stretcher around just below her bottom as if he was dancing with it. "Sit down on our stretcher so we can get you loaded into the back of the truck Miss, we'll take care of you." "GIVE ME SOME PAIN MEDICINE! I NEED IT!" "I can't do that Miss… it's too much of a risk for the baby. The medication crossing the placental barrier can cause terrible side effects," I advised.

"AAHHHHH!" she screamed at the top of her lungs. "I THINK I'M GONNA DIE!" the woman continued. Jeff and I placed her on her side and loosened the stretcher seatbelts — this positioning turned out to give the female patient great relief. Her cries carried on unscrupulously throughout the duration of the transport.

Later finding out that she did end up having a miscarriage (Jeff and I did not disrobe her and evaluate her lady parts), her husband was devastated. He was the messenger we later found out from in passing in the hospital lobby. According to him, his wife didn't want to speak to anyone until further notice. She became intentionally mute due to her loss.

To all the mothers and fathers: this tale goes out to all of the *lost ones*, as I call them. The miscarriages and the abortions. The premature babies that didn't survive. And the small infants who underwent *sudden infant death syndrome*. As your paramedic and friend, my heart goes out to you. I've seen many instances of lost ones. God knows your aches and pains. Losses are simply a part of living. My desire for you as a spiritual advocate is to not get angry at God when negativity intrudes your life. Trust in the Lord and he will give you all the strength that you need. "It only takes faith the size of a mustard seed to move mountains" is what Jesus told us in the Bible. Wellness be with you and your family.

Dearly beloved, avenge not yourselves, but rather give place unto wrath: for it is written, vengeance is Mine; I will repay, saith the Lord. Therefore if thine enemy hunger, feed him; if he thirsts, give him drink: for in so doing thou shalt heap coals of fire on his head. Be not overcome of evil, but overcome evil with good.
Romans 12:19 – 21

#91

Misery Loves Company

Paramedic Pointer» *Interested in learning all about medications? Ever came across an unknown pill? Ever wondered what all those orange prescription bottles actually treated when you saw someone with a handful of them? Drugs.com is an amazing resource for medications; they even have a pill identifier. Happy hunting!*

Each career has its luxuries. A luxury that I personally enjoy as a paramedic is the minimal amount of drama to deal with from coworkers. For the most part, I have one partner, which equates to one person's personality to mesh with. Even still, the truth remains, that misery loves company. Everyone has workplace drama they deal with, no matter what job one has. A partner from my past consistently slandered a lieutenant or chief's name as soon as they left the room. He would snarl and complain the second he disagreed with something from a supervisor and call them names in the process. These kinds of behaviors force one to assume that a person with that character will inevitably do the same to *you*.

One shift, my regular partner having called out sick, left me working with a time bomb waiting to explode. Her name was Ruby and she was as sweet as could be — that was until she, her self, was put in a compromising position.

Ruby got called to headquarters for a meeting with the chiefs about a particular call she ran. The meeting ended in her getting reprimanded, for there was debate about her timeliness in identifying a heart attack in a chest pain patient who died. I was asked to take a seat in the lobby. 20 minutes or so went by and the meeting door opened, signifying the cessation of her disciplinary meeting. I couldn't believe how far she decided to reach to throw some negativity my way. There had been a challenging test our agency decided to give all the county's paramedics — an assessment many did poorly on. Ruby chose to question whether they were going to give me that particular test or not that exact day. She pulled the trigger when I walked in the chief's office to say my goodbyes, extending professionalism as it should have been.

"Are you all going to give Lorenzo his test today? One of the chiefs told me that he was supposed to give Lorenzo the assessment today, but I haven't heard anything else about it," she said, disrupting the complete silence in the office. The three chiefs glanced over their shoulders, displaying looks of confusion. An awkward silence swept the room, Ruby stood in the center looking for someone to break the silence. "Uhhh… I was just wondering because that's what I heard…" she continued. One chief spun completely around in his computer chair to face Ruby; he said, "No… we're not exactly concerned with that right now. Whatever your district chief said is up to *him* to follow through with." Ruby, trying her best to keep a neutral facial expression, quickly exited the room. "Have a good weekend", I said to the three chiefs before exiting the conference room/office.

Round two of Ruby's attempts came when our immediate district chief met us halfway to our station in a vacant parking lot to drop off supplies we needed. "How did your meeting go? Well, I hope," he said with a worrisome look on his face. "It went okay… I still have my job… I'm so pissed at myself… hey are you giving Lorenzo his assessment today?" she said trying to quickly change the subject. Mind you, I'm sitting right next to her in the driver seat of the ambulance cab. "Really, you're bringing this up again?" I thought to myself. "And with no apparent discretion that I see exactly what you're trying to do," I continued to think. "No I don't think I'll be giving Lorenzo that assessment today... I've got so much running around to do," the district chief answered. Ruby remembered from she and I's morning breakfast talk that today was my last shift before five weeks of vacation. "... Well today is his last shift before vacation... you won't see him again for over a month!" she exclaimed.

"Is that right, Lorenzo?" my district chief asked. "Yes," I replied. "... Welp... looks like you have to take the test when you get back!" he said with a huge smile on his face. I could almost feel the temperature of Ruby's blood boiling after our district chief closed the ambulance door and got into his county SUV. Her efforts amounted to nothing. She tried with all her might to redirect the bad juju on to someone else— that particular person being me. I don't believe she had it out for me specifically; I just happened to be the closest person to her she could try to push under the water instead of drowning all by herself, so to speak.

Workplace drama is inevitable—don't allow it to destroy your *own* character by way of irrational impulses. Not everyone will be fond of you and some, as you've seen, will gladly try to direct negative energy on to you. Take the punches as they come, but always conduct yourself so that you can maintain posture. Also, remember that when you're working, God is watching, and he sheds blessings on those who turn the other cheek and strive forward.

Verily, verily, I say unto you, if a man keep My word, he shall never see death. **John 8:51**

#92

Fallen Hero

Paramedic Pointer» *What happens when someone dies? An investigation by the coroner and the police department take place to determine whether suspicious activity was involved, or "foul play". If suspected, the body is taken in for an autopsy. If it is deemed a natural death, then the body is picked up by a mortician and taken to a funeral home (chosen by next of kin).*

CJ, a charismatic black man from Atlanta, Georgia trained me during my initial days out on the street as a medic. He had a thick country accent that took some getting used to — what with it being attached to a black man instead of a white country singer — the normal package I saw that kind of accent come with. CJ taught me many things including: drug calculation methods, starting IVs, effective CPR, critical thinking, etc. He saved many lives and taught me how to do the same; he's responsible for much of my success as a paramedic.

We responded to a trailer park one night filled with nothing but lower class white people for an assault. A Caucasian man came out of left field while we were on scene of that call and yelled, "Get outta here… we don't want your kind around here!" referring to CJ's dark brown complexion. CJ didn't skip a beat on his patient care and attentiveness to the issue at hand. That's the level of character CJ possessed. Always showing positivity to everyone around him, he never let negativity faze him. CJ was into motorcycles — he drove a motorcycle as a primary means of transportation. There wasn't a day when CJ got caught without his racing jacket when he showed up for duty.

The last thing on his mind was the possibility that he would become a patient so soon. At the young age of 33, CJ died in an accident on the highway while he was driving along. Life deals us such peculiar hands at times — one shift CJ was training me, the next shift he was dead. The purpose behind me telling the unfortunate tale of CJ's death is that you think twice, possibly, about the ones who are in your life.

No man or woman can predict the time, place or manner in which they will die. Therefore, we should never shortchange anyone of the love, hospitality and grace they deserve because God does the same for us. It's pure selfishness to not return the same favor to others around us via our *words*. Via our *actions*. Via our *gifts*. Is any grudge really worth holding? Is any ego *really* worth feeding? Is any unnecessary self-centeredness worth employing at the expense of someone else's feelings being damaged? More importantly, the Bible tells us that no one can predict the hour Jesus Christ will return, so I'd like to extend the idea of not taking your *soul* for granted either. We can do this by giving our lives to God and living for him. Then, when Christ judges us, he will see our names in the book of life — the most important book of all.

But my God shall supply all your needs according to his riches in glory by Christ Jesus. **Philippians 4:19**

#93

Too Much Pressure

Paramedic Pointer» *Diet, weight and stress—to name a few— are all factors that affect blood pressure. You can monitor your blood pressure by buying a manual BP cuff or even an automatic. Or, you can simply check it at your grocery store whenever you do your grocery shopping. Monitoring your blood pressure is a simple commitment that will help to avoid future problems. Look out for yourself!*

It's been said that pressure busts pipes when there's enough of it. The saying is another way of communicating that things will fold under the correct circumstances. Cookies will crumble; that sort of thing. A nonliteral example is how we all witnessed the defeat of the Panthers in the 2016 Super Bowl. Defenders were coming from everywhere, causing the talented and elusive quarterback Cam Newton to perform below the level it took to win. I told everyone that he hadn't seen the level of pressure the Denver Broncos placed on teams, being ranked at number one for defense. No one believed my prediction until they saw the Broncos win with their own eyes. It all came down to *pressure*. Pressure is a great force. It distorts things. It causes backup and inversely, the flushing out of even a congested jam. The 2016 Super Bowl example was more of an allegorical reference to the previous phrase I provided regarding pressure.

In a more literal sense, blood vessels are directly affected by pressure — blood pressure. If high enough, one can have a stroke; If too low, one can pass out or lose their pulse altogether. What happened with this particular patient was all about both pressure and time. If you ask him, I'm sure he'll tell you he's glad EMS showed up when they did.

The average sized Caucasian man paced back and forth in his house with his palm to his bald head. Well, he wasn't technically 100% bald; he had a horseshoe of hair to be exact. "Thank God you guys came so fast! I'm freaking out here!" he exclaimed. "I've got the worst headache in the world! It started about 15 minutes ago," he said as he spontaneously wiped his nose. Blood stained his white long sleeve shirt cuff. His shirt was a business shirt, the kind one wears with suit and tie. Blood began to trickle down his nostrils onto his mustache — Jeff and I quickly attached our blood pressure cuff to obtain a reading. "240/120!" Jeff announced as soon as he deflated the BP cuff. Our patient's extremely high blood pressure caused the terrible headache and nosebleed — now it had become evident based off of the numbers.

Jeff applied oxygen to the patient, who sweated more profusely by the second. Anxiety filled the patient's body and exited via his pores in the form of sweat. "Call for a *labetalol* order," I directed Jeff. I began to draw up the medication, a drug made for lowering blood pressure. "The Doc says let him have it!" Jeff said with a stern look on his face. His sentence didn't even come out of his mouth all the way when I began to push the drug. 3 to 5 minutes later, our patient felt a heavy load lifted. "Much better!" he cried. "Give me a repeat on the vital signs, please," I requested of my partner Jeff. "180/90!!" Jeff shouted. "That's a heck of a lot better than the initial reading!" I said. "Yeah... It *feels* a lot better than the prior reading as well!" muttered our patient. "Thank you guys so much for helping me out... it felt like my head was a ticking time bomb getting ready to explode!"

A lovely nurse took report at the ER regarding his elevated blood pressure. "So he's completely stable right now?" she questioned. "... For now at least... when we first made contact with him his pressure was high enough for a stroke, so he'll need close monitoring." —KSSHHH!! "Medic 16, have you made patient transfer yet? We've got a call we want to drop on you!" the female dispatcher advised. Jeff and I darted out of the ER to do it all again. "Thanks again!" our patient's voice diminished as we grew further from his hospital room. There wasn't any time for a proper farewell on our part.

They that trust in the Lord shall be as Mount Zion, which cannot be removed, but abideth forever. **Psalm 125:1**

#94

Hazy Malaise

Paramedic Pointer» Blood is a specialized body fluid that has four components: plasma (carries blood cells), red blood cells (carries oxygen around the body), white blood cells (fights infection and builds immune system), and platelets (forms clots when you get a cut).

Common sense took a backseat on this particular night. If this patient didn't have a neck he would have forgotten his head — that's how forgetful our patient seemed to have been. 10:30 PM crept up on us rather swiftly this shift. We found ourselves having a late dinner, interrupted by our station alarm. Shortly after, a five-story stair climb stood between my partner Jeff, me and the patient. A lofty condominium is where our call resided. Everything as far as the condominium exterior was plush, cocaine white.

"What number was the unit we were looking for again?" I asked Jeff. "Number 502," he replied. Holding on to one side each, we pushed the stretcher down a hallway until we got to unit number 502. A quick glance over the railing opposite to the unit doors revealed nothing but what could be a long drop down to a brutal, traumatic death. "Man… we're wayyy up", I said to Jeff before turning towards the patient's front door. The glass encasement door was shut, but the interior wooden door had been left wide open. I opened the door gently and stepped inside. "PARAMEDICS! PARAMEDICS!

ANYBODY HOME?!" "… Come this way," a soft old voice said from a back room.

"Hello there…" I began as we made it into the patient's bedroom. "What's your issue tonight, Sir?" I questioned. Taking a second to formulate a response, the patient answered, "Something is just not right… my entire body feels weak." Peering around the room briefly for orange prescription bottles, I saw none in sight. A patient's medications are usually a decent indicator of their current dilemma. "How long have you been feeling this way?" "… Oh ever since I swallowed my pills about an hour ago… since then, I've felt really tired." The elderly Caucasian man grabbed a bed pillow and placed it in his lap for his own personal comfort. "Do you have any other complaints outside of feeling tired?" I asked. "Nope… nope. Can't say that I do."

"What were the names of the pills and where are they?" "… In the bathroom on the counter… it starts with an A, but it may start with a B." He appeared to be slightly disoriented, so I asked him a few questions while Jeff sought out the pill bottle in the bathroom. "Can you tell me what city we are in?" Fail. "How about what day of the week it is?" Second failure. "Okay, how about the current president of the United States?" I asked the final question. "Uhh… you know… I'm not sure," the patient said, giving me a blank stare. "His mentation is definitely out of sync," I explained to Jeff as he returned with the orange pill bottle. Handing it to me, Jeff said, "This explains it all." On the bottle, the white label wrapping around it completely, read: *Ambien*. Ambien is a drug prescribed for insomnia. And further, I read that his prescription had been filled earlier that day. The quantity of pills given when filled was 20. I'll let you take a wild guess on how many pills were in the prescription bottle. Here's the answer: *none*. Not even one. Not even a half of a pill. But geez, to think that you wouldn't feel strange or the least bit tired doesn't quite add up — especially when you're the one ingesting the surplus of sleeping pills!

For the Lord giveth wisdom: out of His mouth cometh knowledge and understanding. He layeth up sound wisdom for righteous: He is a buckler to them that walk uprightly. **Proverbs 2:5 – 7**

#95

Delierium Tremens

Paramedic Pointer» *Cortisol is a hormone that stimulates most body cells to increase their energy production.*

In the initial days of being a medic out on the road — and when I say initial I mean literally the first official week — one can surprise you. This was a time when I was shadowing a very smart medic at my first agency. During this time frame, I had not yet seen all of the haphazard conditions patients can present with when you pick them up. So this tale is being told to recognize just how craziness can catch you *unexpectedly*. But hey, you gotta get broken in somehow don't you? At some point, one has to get *thrown to the wolves,* as the saying goes. I'm not sure if there's ever a right time per se, but today was an eye opening experience, to say the least. Even today, I'm not a fan of transporting drunken, bum patients to the hospital, especially when they aren't causing any grief in the community. But something was different about this guy. I found that out soon after we rolled up on him lying on the sidewalk in the middle of the night.

"What's your name, brother?" I asked him as I made a loud plop with my boots after jumping out of the ambulance. "Brandon… I need your help man! My body is bugging out from these withdrawals!" "What drugs were you on?" I inquired. With veins popping out of his head and neck, he answered in a frantic tone, "crack and alcohol… I'm an alcoholic and a habitual crack user bro!" "How old are you, my man?" "27 in December," he replied. Tonight was a November sky. "Help me up brother!" the patient urged with his bulging eyes and serpent like tongue that he kept slipping in and out of his mouth like a snake does, but on fast forward. His body twitched violently and involuntarily. One could have mistaken him to be experiencing seizures, the twitching was so bad. Snatching him up off the ground using one hand, he was then able to make it to the ambulance with assistance.

He wouldn't tolerate our simple measures to evaluate his general stability. He ripped the blood pressure cuff off. He tore the monitor wires away from his chest and threw them on the ambulance floor. It was a wonder how we even got him to sit on the stretcher. Brandon began knee jerking and thrusting his head back into the stretcher's head cushion. He let his tongue hang flaccid out of his mouth and shook his head from side to side in a fit of rage, or better yet, *delirium*. And that's exactly what all this madness is referred to as. Delirium tremens is a severe form of alcohol withdrawal and sometimes a withdrawal from other substances. Brandon digressed into hallucinations too, believing that a flock of birds were antagonizing him with sharp, metallic beaks inside the truck.

"Get them away! Get them away!" Brandon yelled for his life. It wasn't until Jeff and I injected him with *lorazepam* and *thiamine* that Brandon cooled his jets. But as we all know: massive amounts of alcohol consumption breed a full bladder. "I've gotta pee guys!" Brandon said. We ignored his mumbling; it was so distorted at this point that we figured he'd fall asleep for the remaining five minutes of the transport. "I've gotta Pee! Can you guys let me out?!" "No, brother… you're gonna have to hold it." What did this fella think? We were gonna let him out to take a leak in the shoulder of the roadway? "Let me out! I've got a pee!" the man yelled. "We can't allow that Sir… I'm sorry." A few moments passed before I reached up into the cabinet to grab a vomit bag for him to urinate in.

By then it was already too late. Brandon was turned on his side with his junk hanging out, enjoying a long, drawn out release of urine. He didn't even have the decency to aim for the trashcan in his line of sight. All over the ambulance floor, the urine accumulated. Jeff had us stopped at a red light so the back end — where Brandon and I were — was tilted down, causing Brandon's urine to pool in the rearmost corners of the truck. That is, until we hit a patch of bumps in the road! I sat in the captain's chair with my feet raised up in the air — trying earnestly to avoid the small wave pool of pee. "I didn't sign up for this!" I thought. "No one told me I'd be dodging someone's bodily fluids like this!" And do you think Brandon gave a crap? He had his eyes closed, cherishing the flow he had going on to my ambulance floor. He even let out a continuous moan of relief while he was at it. I pondered trying to disrupt him some sort of way but what was I going to do? Attack the guy while he had his business out in the open? Yeah, that would've been fun!

Arrival to the ER premises gave me a rush of joy. Jeff released the residual air from the rear of the ambulance, causing the back end to drop; out poured all of the rank urine upon opening the rear ambulance doors. Brandon was knocked out. We wheeled him into the hospital after we covered him up with a blanket — his pants were still down. And boy did I dread the mere thought of cleaning up the ocean of leftover pee. In the rear of the truck waited a yellowish coated floor. Trying to stay positive through it all, I turned to Jeff and cracked a smile. "You smell that Jeff?" I facetiously questioned. "How could I not Lorenzo... what do you mean?" My response with a big grin: "lemony fresh."

And whatsoever we ask, we receive of Him, because we keep His commandments, and do things that are pleasing in His sight.
1 John 3:22

#96

Find Your Why

Paramedic Pointer» *Passion + Service = Purpose (a practical equation to apply when searching for meaning in your everyday work and life. Don't forget to pray as well)*

Where would you like to make a difference in the world? What could you envision being worth your time? Ask yourself these questions, but more importantly, answer these questions with *no holds barred*. Also, as much as it is important to know what you are going to do in life, it's equally important to know *why*. Countless great contributors were able to do so by way of knowing why they indulged in their craft. Rod Stewart, a rock 'n roll Hall of Fame musician, said he writes and performs music, first of all, because he loves it. Stan Lee had many years of barely making any profit on his *Marvel* superheroes before he blew up and became established. He said that it was his love for the craft that kept him going in his early struggling years. His advice was to indulge yourself in something that you love. In *Made In America* by Sam Walton, founder of Walmart, Mr. Walton reveals that he did as well as he did because from as far back as he could remember, he loved to sell things.

During an interview, Michael Jackson was asked, "How do you create music so efficiently?" His reply was, "When I'm not creating I become down and out — depressed really." Can you see the point I'm getting at? A *love* for the craft may be the reason why you indulge in what you will, and that's perfectly fine. But no matter what you're doing, know *why* you've chosen what you've chosen.

I deem it safe to say that we'd all fancy making large amounts of money. I'm the last person to advise one to ignore making great money, but too many people hate their jobs and find themselves unfulfilled because the only thing they had in mind in school was, "What career pays the best?" My freshman year of college I attended a private institution, studying business management. My reasoning behind it, like many freshmen students with no real life experience, was that it *sounded good*. But then I got to thinking, "Is a business suit and a cubicle really the environment for me?" I enjoy being physical and having autonomy. And I genuinely want to help people who need it. This ran me right into the world of EMS. My sophomore year, I enrolled in paramedic school and got a degree in emergency medical services.

Another reason I chose to become a paramedic is because it reminded me of a ministry. I figured God could use me to help others in the most literal sense. Since my decision to play street doctor, I've been able to impact hundreds of people's lives, seeing wonderful results in all my labor. So I encourage you to be an individual of reason. To take pride in the service you provide to others. We are all made in God's image, everything we do is to reflect and honor his glory. So what is your *love*? What is your *why*? Find it and never let it go.

Evening, and morning, and at noon, will I pray, and cry aloud: and He shall hear my voice. **Psalm 55:17**

#97

PTSD

Paramedic Pointer» *If you ever suffer from PTSD look into EMDR, or eye movement desensitization and reprocessing. Medics, to name one group, have benefited from this therapy immensely. If it can work with us, with all the stress we get inflicted with, it can work for you as well.*

Walking from my car to my apartment front door one morning after coming off duty, I passed a gentleman sitting in a chair with his legs crossed. He took a puff on his cancer stick and said, "Good morning neighbor, just getting off from work?" "You guessed it," I replied. "Hey what do you do anyway? What kind uniform is that?" It was Jesus (pronounced hey-Zeus), the retired military veteran who lived across the hall. "I'm a paramedic." "Oh is that right? Did you know you can get a check for Post-Traumatic Stress Disorder? I did anyway," he said as he readjusted himself in the lawn chair and looked away. "No I don't need that, I'm fine." Jesus squinted his eyes at me and took another puff on his cigarette and said, "You *will* need it, my friend. That kind of work wears on you overtime you know… trust me."

"Well what about you, do you collect a check for PTSD?" "No, I use to though… now I self-medicate," he exclaimed, holding up his cigarette with two fingers and a shiny tin beer can in his other hand. "I'll keep that information in mind," I told Jesus as I entered my apartment. Jesus held up his beer can once more with his eyes closed and said, "cheers."

Policeman, nurses, paramedics, firemen and military personnel are at great risk for PTSD what with the line of work they are in. Constant tragedies are part of the everyday work environment. But PTSD can happen to *anyone*, which is why I found this tale worth visiting. I learned from a traumatized paramedic that there is an incredible therapy for those individuals that suffer from PTSD. And he's a qualified victim indeed. This particular medic was on a routine medical call when he found himself in an unexpected scuffle, leaving him with stab wounds. His aggressor impaled a knife into his back multiple times. After the altercation, the involved paramedic found it extremely difficult to function mentally — he took a leave of absence from work with his department.

But luckily, he found a therapist who gave him treatment he described as *voodoo magic*. He had gone to two other therapists that weren't much help at all, according to him. He had lost confidence in recovering from loss of sleep, flashback trauma and general mental instability and grief. The treatment he received was called EMDR or, eye movement desensitization and reprocessing. In short, it's a methodology of going back to the event and accepting what has happened through various techniques/exercises. I found his testimonial valuable to share for those of you who may incur such mental trauma or have already incurred something that spawned something as serious as PTSD. Be safe out there at all times and keep in mind that you can't always control what happens to you. As for EMDR, there are plenty of resources online that unveil the entire process for your liking.

For if ye forgive men their trespasses, your heavenly Father will also forgive you. **Matthew 6:14**

#98

Heat stroke Heather

Paramedic Pointer » *If There is suspicion of a heat stroke, removal of the patient from that environment is optimal.*

Florida's alias, "the sunshine state" could have been renamed "the sizzling state" today due to 95° plus weather temperatures. My partner Jeff and I's bottle of water had quickly began to sweat and had it not been for us being in a well air-conditioned ambulance, we both would have been drenched in sweat as well. I feared that the ambulance's rubber wheels were going to melt because invisible steam was radiating from the lava hot pavement as we sped down the road on the way to an unconscious female, according to our dispatch notes. The invisible steam I speak of is the steam that makes looking off into the distance blurry on a hot day such as this one. A combination of our driving speed, steam coming from the pavement and the general temperature outside made the expression "burning rubber" come alive. As we bent the corner, we even saw on the curb a bare foot child jumping up and down in efforts to get his mother to pick him up. This was just more confirmation of how the sun was scorching the concrete. Moments later our patient became evident to Jeff and I. Out in the open sun, just baking on the sidewalk was a middle-aged woman sprawled out on the ground. We hopped out of the ambulance and grabbed our stretcher.

On every call we preload the stretcher with three different bags: the cardiac monitor, medical kit and airway bag. Since each call differs, we may bring more or less than these three bags. On this particular call, we cleared the cot of the three bags so that we could immediately place our patient onto the gurney and load her into the ambulance where it was much cooler. For those that are unfamiliar with heatstroke, it is of high importance to quickly remove the patient from the hot environment. Once we picked our unconscious patient up and placed her onto the stretcher, we loaded her into our truck to assess her. She had a pulse and was breathing for starters, signifying that we were not dealing with a clinically dead patient. She was unconscious. Her skin was hot to the touch and there was no mistaking that she was incoherent. I started an IV while Jeff grabbed a few ice packs to help her cool down. We gave fluids through her IV line and placed the cold packs (ice packs) under her armpits, on her neck and in the groin area. Minutes after our initial interventions, she awoke and was confused about where she was.

"What's your name?" I abruptly asked. "I'm Lorenzo and this is my partner Jeff, we picked you up off of the sidewalk a few moments ago... The sun was frying you like an omelet. We'll be your paramedics for today". "I'm Heather", the woman responded. "What's the last thing you remember doing?" Jeff asked. "...Ummm... I... Was just coming from Burger King on my way to Family Dollar", Heather replied. Mind you, Burger King and Family Dollar were literally right across the street from one another which meant it took Heather not much time at all to be acutely affected by the unforgiving Florida sun. It didn't help that she was dehydrated as well. Her tongue was not the usual healthy pinkish red color, rather it was mostly white, which is a sign of being dehydrated. Heather told us that she had not drank anything in hours, ordering a milkshake instead of water or another beverage while at Burger King. With more and more fluid being delivered into her body, Heather was starting to look like a new person. Her skin, which was extremely pale when we first made contact with her, was now a more vibrant, healthy color that reflected good circulation. Preparing to leave the scene en route to the hospital, Heather asked, "Can I have a blanket...? I'm cold". I grabbed a blanket out of our cabinet and covered her with it. Our methods of rapid cooling had worked! Between removing her from the sun, turning the air conditioner on high with the temperature as low as it could go and inundating her with ice packs, we had successfully cooled Heather off!

Thankfully it resulted in a positive outcome— the kind of outcome we paramedics always strive for. Arriving at the hospital, we gave patient report to the nurse and obtained a signature for transfer of care. Patient report is nothing more than reporting what the patient's problem was, how we fixed it and other pertinent findings such as a patient's medical history, allergies to medications, medications currently taken etc. Also, we must always obtain a signature from the hospital facility representative because when we transfer a patient, the liability then goes to the receiving hospital. We advised Heather to stay hydrated and bid her a farewell, wishing her no more 911 emergencies in the future.

Therefore if any man be in Christ, he is a new creature: old things are passed away; behold, all things are become new. 2 Corinthians 5:17

#99

Snakes On An Ambulance

Paramedic Pointer» The small intestine in adults is a long and narrow tube about 7 meters (23 feet) in length. The large intestine is so called because it is larger in diameter. However, it is shorter than the small intestine, only about 1.5 meters feet (5 feet) in length. That should take care of the childhood myth that claims the intestines can span for miles.

America's symbol for healthcare and medicine used on ambulances, hospitals and clinics is a winged staff with two serpents entwined on it. This symbol is called the *caduceus* and it can be located on the back cover of this very book. The word caduceus refers to an ancient Greek or Roman herald's wand associated with healing. In ancient Greece and ancient Roman times it was believed that serpents had healing powers and the gift of immortality due to the shedding of skin — a perceived renewal of the body. It is a widely accepted legend that the Greek God Hermes was walking along with his rod one day to find two snakes at war.

He allegedly placed his staff between the two serpents in a beguiled manner and they entwined on it in peace. It is said that the two serpents represent polar opposites (i.e. male and female, yin and yang). The United States has adopted this symbol as a universal representation of medicine. However, many sources say that the caduceus medical symbol was incorrectly chosen out of ignorance and confusion coupled with pseudo-research. Altogether, the use of the caduceus is believed to be an erroneous selection because before the caduceus was the *rod of Asclepius*, another Greek God in Greek mythology who was a deity associated with healing and medicine.

The rod of Asclepius has a single serpent entwined on it, as opposed to the double serpent rod with wings the caduceus symbol has. In Greek mythology, Hermes (holder of the caduceus) was also associated with *commerce*. Both symbols are used, the caduceus being surpassingly more used out of the two. Sources say that professional associations often choose the rod of Asclepius because they are more aware of its true meaning, whereas commercial associations use the caduceus symbol due plainly to its better visual appeal. In other words, the caduceus is felt to be more marketable. 1902 marked the initial formal adoption of the caduceus by the Medical Department of the US Army and was added to the uniforms of Army medical officers.

The way of a fool is right in his own eyes: but he that hearkeneth unto counsel is wise. **Proverbs 12:15**

#100

The Secret Within Volunteering

Paramedic Pointer» *Any opportunity could have hidden treasure, don't be so dismissive as to ignore what could very well lie right before you. Assess each opportunity meticulously for its value.*

Allow me to preface this illustration of pro bono labor by saying that if you are the typical minded individual as I once was, then you feel that volunteering is for suckers and people that have absolutely nothing better to do with their time. After all, "Bills have got to be paid. Life isn't free!" you say. "How foolish would it be to give away free labor *and* time! What a crime what with all the precious wages and energy lost!" you cry. There is a secret behind the act of volunteering that exists for your own benefit; I recognized it shortly after being forced to volunteer in college and after college during the pursuit of my EMS career.

The first undesirable instance of volunteering came during hours of time spent at an assisted living facility for the elderly. My second volunteer experience came when I had to spend six months volunteering in a firehouse in order to keep my firefighter certification valid. It was not until after my second experience that the epiphany came to me, and even then it wasn't a self-proclaimed epiphany. It was articulated to me rather eloquently by a successful businessman. His message resonated with me and so now I find it necessary to pass the wisdom on to my valued reader, especially the reader who has yet to come into his or her career. The person pondering which profession to partake in or even one who currently has a career, but is looking to change their profession, could benefit greatly from this truth.

The secret within volunteering is that one is privileged, in a sense, to taste before he or she swallows. Specifically, one is able to exercise a *trial run* before subscribing. Colleges present a four-year degree system that tells you to study hard and long on subjects you personally handpick to obtain a degree in. No one can argue that knowledge is inevitably required to function properly in a vocation or practice of any kind, at least on a professional level. But what about hands on experience? Though reading something can be fascinating, physically doing it can be in great opposition.

Suppose you study for four years, or however long you decide, only to find out that you deplore the actual job itself? Then what? You get the honor of riding out a bad decision, in all its misery, or simply start over again, realizing that you wasted precious time? Make your decisions wisely, fellow readers, and consider using volunteering as a beneficial opportunity. Look at it as a test run to something you are seriously considering. It's a wise investment as opposed to the nightmare of fruitless efforts.

www.ingramcontent.com/pod-product-compliance
Lightning Source LLC
Chambersburg PA
CBHW022052210326
41519CB00054B/314